# HIGH BLOOD
# PRESSURE

# HIGH BLOOD PRESSURE

*What causes it*
*How to tell if you have it*
*How to control it for a longer life*

FRANK A. FINNERTY, Jr., M.D.

*and* SHIRLEY MOTTER LINDE

*The David McKay Company, Inc., New York*
IN COOPERATION WITH
*Pavilion Publishing Company, Inc., New York*

*Second Printing, March 1975*

HIGH BLOOD PRESSURE: *What causes it, How to tell if you have it, How to control it for a longer life*

*Copyright © 1975 by*
*Shirley Motter Linde and Frank A. Finnerty, Jr., M.D.*

*Library of Congress Catalog Card Number: 74–83690*
*ISBN: 0–679–50512–1*
MANUFACTURED IN THE UNITED STATES OF AMERICA

*This book has been written to bring the story of high blood pressure to the public. It has been reviewed by the National High Blood Pressure Education Program, the American Heart Association, the American Medical Association, the National Medical Association, and the Citizen's Committee for the Treatment of High Blood Pressure.*

*The book tells you what high blood pressure is, how you can tell if you have it, and what specific things your doctor and you can do to treat it and prevent its complications.*

# *Preface*

This is a most timely book. It comes at a time when we know what the essential problem in hypertension is; we have several drugs available to treat it; and we know what those drugs will do.

The therapy available now, and detailed in these pages, will save lives. Deaths due to hypertension, hypertensive heart disease, and stroke are decreasing. This decrease— and the decrease can be seen in each age group—is apparent in the data routinely compiled by the National Office of Vital Statistics. But these same data also reveal how much is yet to be accomplished. Sixty thousand people in the United States still die each year from hypertensive disease. Unnecessary, preventable death is always a waste. In both the young and the middle-aged—people with families to support, children to raise, and a wife or husband to cherish —premature, preventable death is a tragedy.

"Let us grow old together" is a Jewish prayer all too infrequently heard these days. Yet, it bespeaks an understanding of people and their needs rarely apparent in the plans of social architects or in the minds of most adults.

The economists know some of the fiscal problems of hypertensive disease and premature death. There are no data for the total social costs of this disease. But the medical care costs and the wages lost to cardiovascular disease of all types has been estimated at $19.5 billion per year.

Few people, if given a choice, would choose to die young. Fewer would choose to live out their lives crippled, blind, or unable to think or speak clearly. Yet, this is the fate of many people with high blood pressure. It is a burden doubly hard to bear because it is unnecessary. Most of the complications of hypertension can be prevented in most people. Certainly the appearance of complications can be postponed. And every day lived in health is a day to be cherished.

This book tells how to obtain such days. If it did only this, and only for people with high blood pressure, it would be well worthwhile. But it does more. And from the point of view of the health of the public in general this *more* may come to be recognized as the critical factor in maintaining health. Here we have a clear statement of what the patient and the physician can do, and must do, together, if the ravages of chronic disease are to be prevented.

If chronic disease, chronic heart disease, hypertensive heart disease, and stroke are to be prevented, the patient, the "apparently" healthy man or woman, must take an active interest in doing so, must play a positive role in seeking medical advice, adhering to instruction, and maintaining prescribed drug regimens. Like a young child whose balloon has burst, the public, the layman, the potential patient must learn that some things cannot be fixed, they can only be prevented.

Where maintenance of health, not just treatment for disease, is the goal, patient and physician must be partners together. That the physician needs special training for his role in this partnership has long been recognized, if not always fully realized. That the healthy patient needs help to play his role adequately has only recently been acknowledged.

This book contains the needed help and advice that people with hypertension must have if they are to be effective partners with their physician in controlling their disease and maintaining their state of health. It only remains for all the people "at risk" to read and to act upon this advice.

THEODORE COOPER, M.D.
*Director, National Heart and Lung Institute*

# *Foreword*

_____

_____

_____

The authors believe that patients have a right to be informed about their medical problems.

This is especially true in the case of patients with high blood pressure, because patients with this disease are called upon to modify their style of living and to take medicine that may in some cases make them temporarily feel less well. Therapy recommended to prevent future consequences can be accepted by a patient only if he understands his disease completely.

This book is designed to educate the public, but the education of physicians will be an important secondary effect. Many doctors educated twenty-five or thirty years ago do not realize the importance of treating hypertension, and therefore tend to ignore elevations of blood pressure which are now known to be significant. An informed patient population requesting that blood pressures be taken will indirectly result in an upgrading of physicians' understanding of hypertension.

The authors advise patients to expect that their blood pressure be taken on the occasion of any contact with the health-care system, whether through a dentist, an ophthalmologist, or a gynecologist. Patients are also encouraged to ask for the numerical value of their blood pressure and to inquire about the need for treatment. An informed patient will not accept statements such as "It's a little bit high"; "It's normal"; "You needn't worry about it."

This book goes far beyond a discussion of hypertension alone, however. It outlines a program for healthful living. It tells what to do about smoking and elevated cholesterol, and gives commonsense advice about diet, exercise, and how to deal with the stresses and anxieties of life.

The writing style is perfectly matched to the purpose of the book. It is conversational, with many topics handled in question-and-answer format, and there are case histories to illustrate specific points. The tone is geared to the reader who wants to learn more than is available in pamphlets but does not have the background to interpret articles in medical textbooks or journals. Familiar, everyday language is used to emphasize points, as for example: "You can be the coolest dude in town and still have high blood pressure."

*High Blood Pressure* is designed to inform the lay public about the prevention of common cardiovascular diseases. The patient with high blood pressure will certainly benefit from the wise and practical advice given here, but the book also contains good medical information for anyone interested in good health.

RICHARD S. ROSS, M.D.
Professor of Medicine; Director,
Cardiovascular Division, Johns Hopkins
Medical Institutions.
President, American Heart Association.

# A Statement by the American Medical Association on the Control of Hypertension*

———————————

———————————

———————————

The National Heart and Lung Institute, under the leadership of Theodore Cooper, M.D., has launched a nationwide program to inform the public about hypertension, and to engage the medical profession in a rigorous effort to screen all patients for the disease. The American Medical Association independently established a special committee to review the problem and to outline a series of proposals for effective action. It is clear from its initial study that two major themes must be struck: First, all patients must have their blood pressures taken (by ophthalmologists, dermatologists, orthopedists, psychiatrists, dentists, school nurses, and family planning counselors); that is, whenever a patient reports for any type of examination or counsel, the blood pressure must be taken. Second, if an elevated blood pressure is observed, active treatment should be begun immediately and must be sustained. . . .

All patients can be treated, and almost all will respond with a lowering of blood pressure. Getting across that relatively uncomplicated message is probably one of the most important steps of both public and professional education.

* Reprinted from the *Journal of the AMA,* April 16, 1973.

An informed and insistent effort by all physicians might well have an extraordinary impact on the eventual toll that untreated hypertension extracts from those who have the disease.

MORTON D. BOGDONOFF, M.D.
Chairman, AMA
Committee on Hypertension

# Acknowledgments

The authors wish to express sincere appreciation to the following organizations and individuals for their help as we gathered and prepared the material contained in this book.

American College of Cardiology
American Health Foundation
American Heart Association
American Medical Association
W. A. Baum Co.
Alton Blakeslee
Blue Cross–Blue Shield
Morton D. Bogdonoff, M.D.
CIBA Pharmaceutical Company
Citizens for the Treatment of High Blood Pressure
Theodore Cooper, M.D.
Charles L. Curry, M.D.
Edward Freis, M.D.
Georgetown University
Georgia Heart Association
Louise S. Hauenstein, Ph.D.
John H. Laragh, M.D.
Mary Lasker
William E. Learnard
*Medical Opinion*

Menninger Foundation
Merck & Co.
Metropolitan Life Insurance Co.
Campbell Moses, M.D.
National Association for Mental Health
National Heart and Lung Institute
National High Blood Pressure Education Program
National Medical Association
Helen Neal
Rockefeller University
Richard Ross, M.D.
Science and Medicine Publishing Company
Smith Kline & French
Maurice Sokolow, M.D.
John B. Stokes III, M.D.
Emery Rann, M.D.
University of Michigan

# Contents

_____

_____

_____

# A Message from the Authors

_____

_____

_____

High blood pressure kills more Americans than any other single disease. In fact, it kills more people in the world than cars, cancer, fire, murder, or anything else you can name.

The chances are that one out of five of you (one out of three if you are black or over the age of fifty) has high blood pressure, and at least half of you who have it do not know you have it. You don't know about it because high blood pressure causes absolutely no symptoms until it is too late. The only way to tell if your blood pressure is high is to have it checked.

What makes knowing you have it so important is that effective treatment is available. Frequently, taking a pill a day is all that is needed to control your blood pressure—and controlling blood pressure prevents strokes, heart failure, and kidney failure, which are the complications of high blood pressure.

This is what this book is all about. To give you the straight talk—no holds barred—on what high blood pressure or hypertension really is; to tell you how simple it is to find out if you have it; and, more important, to tell you what you can do about it.

Don't wait until you have a stroke or your heart fails.

Read this book! We have separated the facts from the old wives' tales. Now go find out what your blood pressure is. This book may well save your life!

FRANK A. FINNERTY, JR., M.D.
SHIRLEY MOTTER LINDE

# 1

## The Silent Killer

It was early in 1973. Some 300 people were gathered in a large hotel meeting room in Washington to discuss a vital subject—high blood pressure.

Some of the men there were research scientists, some were doctors in practice. All of them were leaders in medicine, either specialists in high blood pressure and heart disease, or heads of important medical organizations and government departments.

All of them were concerned with the fact that, today, high blood pressure is apparently the number-one killer of the American people—and nothing that really counted was being done about it.

These medical men listened intently as dynamic Dr. Theodore Cooper, director of the government's National Heart and Lung Institute, opened the meeting, outlining how both government and private groups were concerned about high blood pressure as a menacing public health problem.

And they listened again when Elliot Richardson, then Secretary of Health, Education, and Welfare, talked about the need for a crusade. He called high blood pressure a "powerful but insidious enemy."

"It affects the health, the well-being, and the very life of many people," said Mr. Richardson.

"Hypertension [another name for high blood pressure] begins to claim its victims even before they reach adulthood. The threat increases with each additional year of life.

"There are some 23 million Americans—more than one in ten—who now have high blood pressure. Of these, 60,000 die every year as a direct result of their disease. In addition, hypertension is an underlying cause of more than a million heart attacks and strokes which occur annually in this country, killing or making invalids of their victims.

"By any measure," he went on, "it is indeed an understatement to term hypertension one of our foremost health hazards. The problem is compounded by the fact that at least half of the people who have high blood pressure are not even aware of it. Damocles, as he sat at a banquet table in ancient Greece, at least had the advantage of knowing about the sword that hung by a single hair above his head. Yet here, in twentieth-century America, millions of people are sitting or walking around quite unaware that their bodies carry hidden time bombs ticking toward the moment of detonation."

"And," he told the doctors, "a note of tragic irony is added. *Hypertension can be brought under control by proven treatment which is neither unduly hazardous, expensive, or complicated.*"

But despite the fact that we have the medical knowledge and the medicines to treat high blood pressure, Richardson said, they are not being used. *"Millions of our fellow citizens are not getting the full benefit of this medical knowledge and skill."*

This is why we have written this book. To bring to you and others the facts about high blood pressure, to explain to you how it is a killer, and does its damage, how you may have it and not know it. And, most important, to tell you how you can find out what your blood pressure is, and, if you have high blood pressure, what you can do about it.

## *The facts about high blood pressure*

• High blood pressure is *the* major hazard to health in the country today. It is an epidemic.

• High blood pressure is the leading cause of strokes.

• It is the leading cause of heart failure.

• It is the leading cause of kidney failure.

• It is the major cause of death among blacks for sure, and perhaps among whites also.

• It is a major risk factor in heart attacks.

• In fact, high blood pressure is probably *the* leading single risk factor in causing *all* disability and death in the United States and many other countries today.

It kills, directly or indirectly, more people than cancer, than polio, than tuberculosis, or emphysema, or any other disease you can name. It killed more people in 1973 than the Viet Nam War and automobile accidents combined.

And yet, people know almost nothing about high blood pressure. They have no realization of how important and dangerous it is. And the doctors are almost as unconcerned. Listen to these figures.

More than 23 million people in the United States are officially estimated currently to have high blood pressure. But insurance company data suggest that the number is closer to 40 million. In the entire world there may be some half a billion people living day by day with the unknown danger.

Of these, less than 50 percent know that they have high blood pressure.

And less than 10 percent are getting effective treatment! Scary? You know it is. Almost unbelievable.

Furthermore, there's no way to tell whether you have high blood pressure without being checked. You can feel healthy and look terriffic, but you may have been living for years with the hidden time bomb of high blood pressure doing internal damage to your body.

Then one day the symptoms suddenly appear—when damage is already done. Or you may even suddenly blow a gasket and drop dead, never knowing what hit you. There's no way to tell in advance. Imagine a disease with absolutely no symptoms until harm has been done.

That's the bad news about high blood pressure.

### The good news

Now here's the good news.

The good thing about high blood pressure is that you *can* do something about it. It's not like other major diseases such as cancer that are so difficult to control. High blood pressure can be controlled. And the complications it causes—stroke, heart failure, kidney failure, and sudden premature death—*can* be prevented.

You can live a normal life even if you have high blood pressure, as long as you take the medicine that keeps it down.

### It's your choice

You can have high blood pressure and ignore it, taking a chance that serious complications will occur. Or you can take pills to lower blood pressure to certainly prolong life and health.

That's the choice.

First, of course, you have to find out if you have it.

### Know your number

You know your telephone number, you know your house number. You know your social security and licence plate number. You know your weight and height.

But do you know your blood pressure number? Most people don't.

And if you do, do you know whether it is high or considered within the normal range?

This information could save your life.

We'll tell you in this book where you can find out about your blood pressure, even how to measure it at home. And we'll give you the recommendations on how often you should have your blood pressure checked and what the numbers mean when you get them.

### *Another problem—and a paradox*

Detecting hypertension is easy. Recording blood pressure takes less than one minute, and is painless.

Medical treatment is readily available and relatively simple to administer. And there is ample proof that therapy can effectively reduce disability and death.

Yet, we physicians have not succeeded in making any real progress in identifying the millions of people who have hypertension and don't know it. And we are not giving adequate treatment to most of those we have identified.

How can this appalling situation exist? Part of the reason is that most patients with hypertension are completely without symptoms and resist taking medication unless they are truly motivated.

But another large part of the problem is that many physicians do not record blood pressure as a routine part of a patient's visit; or if they do take the pressure they treat only those patients with the more severe elevations of blood pressure. Several studies have shown this.

In Charlottesville, Virginia, Dr. Carlos Ayers found that 80 percent of internists, ob-gyns, and family practitioners took blood pressures routinely on first visits and at least annually thereafter, but only 20 percent of doctors in other specialties did so.

Dr. Edward Frohlich, professor of medicine and director of the division of hypertension at the University of Oklahoma, says, "When we examined the charts of 200 patients admitted to hospitals, we found that one out of every four patients didn't have their blood pressure taken on examination by a doctor."

In Chicago, four researchers—Dr. James A. Schoenberger, Dr. Jeremiah Stamler, Richard B. Shekelle, and Susan Shekelle—found that of patients suffering from high blood pressure, almost 60 percent did not know they had it. And only 11 percent were under proper care, despite the fact that 90 percent of the women and 75 percent of the men had seen their doctors in the preceding two years.

The doctors reported in the Journal of the American Medical Association, "It must be concluded that physicians had never made the diagnosis of hypertension or had deliberately not informed their patients."

Think of the number of people who would immediately be screened if all doctors, including psychiatrists, dermatologists, otolaryngologists, and other specialists would routinely record blood pressures. Any person who visits a physician or any medical facility for any reason should automatically have his blood pressure checked.

Just this year, the American Medical Association came out with a formal statement recommending that a blood pressure measurement be made a part of *every* initial physical examination by *any* physician, no matter what his specialty.

But just recording the blood pressure doesn't solve anything, either. Dr. Stamler, then director of the Chicago Health Research Foundation, also reports that when a large group of men who worked for a utility company were found to have high blood pressure and were referred to their private doctors, one-third were never treated by those doctors. And since the study was a long term study, most of the men had been referred a number of times, year after year, but still were never treated by their doctors.

And in another study, Dr. Schoenberger found that more than half of newly discovered hypertensive patients in the offices of cardiologists and internists were not even given a second appointment!

The message that high blood pressure can be treated and that treating it significantly reduces risk of heart disease, stroke, and early death has obviously not reached the majority of practicing physicians. Indeed, a smaller percentage of hypertensives are being treated today than there were several years ago.

### The other side

There is one other side to the lack of proper treatment: although most physicians know that treatment will help patients with severe high blood pressure, they're not completely convinced that therapy is beneficial to patients with less severe elevations of blood pressure. They don't want to put a patient on lifelong treatment if they're not sure it's going to do him any good.

Now, to be conservative is fine; to be sure that people really need medicine before you give it to them is a basic philosophy of good medicine. But in this case, conservatism has gone too far. Veterans Administration and Public Health studies have documented the benefits of treating patients whose diastolic blood pressure is persistently over 105 mm Hg. People who have this high a pressure and should be getting treatment are not. Maybe we simply haven't gotten the message across to the doctors as yet. In any event, high blood pressure is not being taken seriously enough.

### Medical attitudes

Part of the reason for this is that medical ideas about high blood pressure have been changing. Some thirty years or so ago, doctors thought some degree of high blood pressure was *good* for you, that you needed it to pump blood through arteries that were becoming narrower and harder with age. But now it has been shown that high blood pressure is never good.

Some doctors, however, still are living with the old ideas. In addition, many university centers place the highest priority on the diagnosis of rare forms of high blood pressure and place little emphasis on treatment of the kind that nine out of ten people have. This has led to the routine performance of expensive, sophisticated tests on newly discovered hypertensives. The expense has been a barrier to physician and patient alike, and has frequently delayed institution of effective therapy. Indeed, many patients are only investigated and never treated.

This is exemplified tragically in the true story of a doctor who was one of the important leaders of American medicine, about, in fact, to be put up as the next president of the American Medical Association.

Actually, he was first diagnosed as having high blood pressure some twenty-five years ago when he was a medical student, but there weren't any effective drugs for high blood pressure then, and not much could be done for him. Since he had no symptoms, he more or less forgot about it.

But in the last ten years—after effective drugs for high blood pressure had been discovered and proved effective— he had physical checkups by twelve different internists, all of them friends of his and teaching at different medical centers across the country. Each of them examined him and investigated him fully (special x-rays, every conceivable blood test) but not one treated his high blood pressure.

Last year, the doctor had a severe attack of high blood pressure on his vacation, and his pressure soared up seventy points above normal limits. This time, a doctor paid attention to his hypertension and treated it with medication. The medicine brought his pressure down, so after a while he foolishly decided to try going without it. Then he had a stroke, with irreversible brain damage. That was just before he was about to be nominated for AMA president. Several months later he died.

The story—hard to believe, but true—points up just how much high blood pressure is being ignored, not only by the public, but by the medical profession itself.

## The hypertension problem

What can be done about this? Physicians must be re-educated to consider that strokes, kidney failure, and heart failure are all preventable complications of hypertension and, therefore, that all patients with hypertension, even mild hypertension, should be treated.

If physicians would recognize, appreciate, and take advantage of the recent advances in therapy, millions of hypertensives could be brought under care and treatment, and could immediately be given a new lease on life.

## The patient's role

Let's not rest the blame completely on the physician. Patients must also be educated to seek medical care, not just when they feel sick, but in order to stay well.

This program of education is now beginning to move. The National Heart and Lung Institute, the American Heart Association and many others have joined together in a massive drive to get information to the public and to physicians on the need to treat high blood pressure.

Information is being sent out, screening centers are being set up, treatment schedules are being recommended.

But all of these measures, in the end, depend on the patient's willingness to take advantage of them.

*You* must go to a doctor or clinic or a screening center to learn if you have high blood pressure.

*You* must carry through, if your pressure is high, and see your doctor for further evaluation and treatment.

*You* must take your pills every day and follow whatever other advice is given you.

It is only by doing these things that you can assure yourself of as many good years of a good life as possible. For with high blood pressure you *can* still live the good life, *can* do the things you want to do.

In the next chapters we will tell you how to find out whether you need to worry about high blood pressure, and if you have it, what you can do about it.

# 2

# *How to Tell If You Have It*

Bill was an account executive with an advertising agency. He always considered himself in good health, with only a cold or two or a week of flu that might knock him out of work occasionally. He never really thought much about his health; in fact, he considered himself such a superior physical specimen that he never bothered to get a regular physical exam like most of the other men at the office. He was always too busy or had something more important to do with his money—or he simply didn't think about it.

One day he noticed that he was puffing a lot going up stairs, but figured it was just part of getting older. He seemed to be tired all the time, too, didn't have the get-up-and-go he used to. In fact, and this really worried him, he didn't have that same old sex drive, either. As a matter of fact, he had to admit he sometimes simply couldn't have an erection.

The next thing he noticed was that he always seemed to get up in the middle of the night to urinate.

Then one day Bill had to go in for a checkup as a requirement for a new insurance policy. When the doctor sat down to talk to him after all the examinations and tests, it wasn't very good news. Bill's blood pressure was very high and had apparently been taking its toll for years. Now his heart was badly enlarged and was not pumping efficiently, which allowed fluid to back up in the lungs. His kidneys were severely damaged too, working overtime at night trying to rid his body of poisonous substances. It was impossible to assess the condition of all the blood vessels going to his vital organs, but those that could be seen in the back of his eyes showed deterioration—they were old before their time.

What happened to Bill is what can happen to anyone who does not have his blood pressure checked regularly. Because *the truth is that high blood pressure usually doesn't give you any warning.*

Until the damage is done—until complications develop—there really are no symptoms.

If you are beginning to get symptoms similar to Bill's, it means there is beginning to be some blood vessel damage. If there is visual deterioration, dizziness, or headache, blood vessel damage to the brain has probably already occurred. If there is shortness of breath, swelling of the ankles, or chest pain, it may mean there is already some heart damage. If you have trouble going through the night without going to the bathroom two or three times, you may have kidney damage.

### *Are there* any *warnings of high blood pressure?*

Almost never. It is truly a silent disease. Doctors cannot stress enough the point that in the beginning and for many years, sometimes twenty years or more, high blood pressure can be causing terrible internal damage to the body with absolutely no outward signs or symptoms. The housewife, the physician, salesman, teacher, scientist, bus driver, all can go happily about their daily living, never knowing that their blood pressure is dangerously high until symptoms do appear, or they have their pressure measured.

You are aware of how your pulse quickens when you are excited, or frightened. But your blood pressure can go up without your knowing it.

### What about nosebleed?

Occasionally, a severe nosebleed will occur with high blood pressure. But it does not happen often; only a very few of those with high blood pressure actually get a warning nosebleed. And a nosebleed can also arise from many other causes: from something as simple as the dry thin membranes that accompany an allergy or a cold to the fact that you picked your nose and hit a blood vessel.

### What about a red face?

Many people think of a red face or florid complexion as a sure sign of elevated blood pressure. Sometimes it is, but more often not.

A man with a ruddy face can have low pressure. A pasty paleface can have high pressure.

### What about sexual symptoms and general fatigue?

Dr. Theodore Cooper, director of the National Heart and Lung Institute, and Dr. Mitchell Perry, head of one of the government's task forces on high blood pressure were talking about these symptoms one evening after a meeting.

"Often," said Dr. Cooper, "if a patient does have a symptom, it may not seem related to high blood pressure, and the physician may not even take his blood pressure."

"One middle-aged male patient came to a doctor complaining of impotence," Dr. Cooper said. "The first time he saw the patient, the physician found no particular reason for the impotence. But he did not take the blood pressure. On a second visit, he finally did take the pressure, which was very elevated. Once the blood pressure was treated the man's performance was restored."

Of all symptoms, impotence probably brings a patient to the doctor fastest, according to Dr. Perry. But even then he doesn't realize he's not feeling up to par.

"There may be tiredness, lassitude, failure to perform in many ways," said Perry. "I've had many a patient after he's been treated say, 'You know, I didn't really know that I felt bad beforehand, but I feel better now than I've felt for years!' "

## What about headache, dizziness, shortness of breath?

These are typically thought of as symptoms of high blood pressure. And they can be, but usually by the time they appear it means your heart or brain or kidneys have already suffered damage from the elevated pressure. And again, as is true in so many cases, they can be symptoms of other diseases or ailments, quite distinct from high blood pressure.

## And kidney problems?

If you go through the night without urinating, your kidney function is all right. If you have to get up at night to urinate, it may mean you have kidney damage, but not necessarily. It could also mean you have prostate trouble, are pregnant, or that you have been drinking more than a beer or two before going to bed.

And again, it is a late sign; damage has already begun.

## *Heart symptoms?*

If your heart has been affected by your high blood pressure, you may have chest pains. Or, you may have trouble getting your breath when you walk up stairs or run. You may also wake up wheezing in the middle of the night, unable to get your breath unless you sit up or prop your head up on several pillows. You may notice, too, that your shoes are too tight, indicating an accumulation of fluid in your feet and ankles.

You must see your doctor if you have any such symptoms. Only he can properly interpret them.

## *Distended neck veins?*

When the neck veins are noticeably distended, especially when an individual is inhaling, his heart may be "overloaded"—that is, overworked. Symptoms of high blood pressure will often be seen along with the distended veins, but again it is a late sign.

## *How long does it take for these symptoms to appear?*

In some cases, high blood pressure comes on suddenly. In others, it builds up gradually.

In some people, it takes such a severe form that damage can be done in a few months. Others have a milder form that may be hidden for twenty years before heart damage is done, for thirty years before the brain is affected. The best way to avoid damage is to keep track of your blood pressure regularly so that the symptoms never appear.

If you have *any* of these symptoms, see your doctor immediately. The more severe they are, the more urgent it is to see him.

But the point is, don't wait till these symptoms appear. Check your blood pressure now!


### *Are there any early warning signs?*

No. You may simply feel tired and not up to par. Or you may feel in the best of health.

The only way to know if you have high blood pressure is to have it measured.


### *How one doctor's life was saved*

Just how sneaky high blood pressure can be is reflected in the personal story of Dr. B. B. Eddleman, professor of medicine at the University of Alabama School of Medicine. Ten years ago, he was giving a lecture when he suffered a severe nosebleed. He was rushed off to the university's hospital, where the nosebleed was stopped, but a colleague found his blood pressure to be 260/160, a frighteningly high level.

Dr. Eddleman, writing in the magazine *Medical Opinion*, explains that his case of high blood pressure came on suddenly, from a reading of normal pressure in January to the life-threatening level six months later.

But, he said, "While in the hospital I realized that there were symptoms I had ignored over the last few months. In January of 1963 my blood pressure was normal. By March I was having severe headaches that were sometimes accompanied by nausea. I'd had tension headaches before, so I tossed off these signs as insignificant. Looking back, I had another symptom: personality change.

"In the few short months between January and June I

gradually developed a very negative attitude toward almost everything."

His research work in computer diagnosis of the heart suffered as he became less productive.

"I was, in all, a disgruntled individual, and I don't think I was very pleasant with my friends and family. I suppose the headaches or personality change separately might have meant any number of things. But together they offered a clear indication of hypertension, and I sometimes feel a little chagrin that I didn't at least take my own blood pressure during this time."

"Luckily," he adds, "my case of malignant hypertension had tipped itself off by epistaxis [nosebleed], and had developed so suddenly that tests showed little or no kidney damage."

Dr. Eddleman was put on high blood pressure drugs, and is still on them.

"Today my blood pressure is under complete control," he says, "and it's been that way for about the last decade. I suffer no side effects whatsoever, and the drugs I now take offer no impairment in functioning or life style. All symptoms of malignant hypertension have long since disappeared, and while I have little doubt I could come off these drugs, I see no reason to tempt another bout of this hypertension. Once blood pressure was lowered, my personality returned to normal—whatever that may be—and is no longer characterized by the negativism I once felt. I enjoy my family, colleagues, research, and expect to live to a ripe old age."

Dr. Eddleman mentions one ironic note: The day he had the nosebleed he was lecturing on high blood pressure.

But not all of us are as fortunate as Dr. Eddleman. More often than not, high blood pressure carries no warning signal. The best defense against it is periodic recordings of your blood pressure. Should it start to rise, drugs can almost always pull it down again, and that's a ticket for longer life.

# 3

# *Who Gets It?—Age, Race, and Early History*

Anyone can get high blood pressure. It can turn up in a child a few years old, or wait to make its first appearance in that same person eighty years later.

It strikes either sex, people of any race or nationality, of all degrees of economic, educational, and professional status. Anybody can get it.

But there are variations in susceptibility within groups, variations that have to do with age and sex. There are also racial differences. Family histories are important in predicting the possibility of high blood pressure. And how you live. Some people are more likely to get high blood pressure than others. Some are affected by it more than others.

For example, if you are a man over age fifty, the chances are one in three that you already have it. If you are black, you are even more likely to have it than if you are white. If you are on birth control pills, you are more likely to have it than if you are not.

This chapter will tell you about all these differences and will help you look at your own personal profile to determine what the chances are that you might be affected by high blood pressure.

### At what age does high blood pressure usually begin?

The average age at which high blood pressure begins is in the thirties, probably earlier in blacks. However, it can occur at any age, and has been found in children aged four.

And it is dangerous at any age. If you begin to get high blood pressure at the age of thirty, and you don't treat it, you will, according to the law of averages, probably die of its complications between the ages of fifty to fifty-five.

### Why do we think of it as being a disease of older age?

High blood pressure is thought of as a disease that strikes older people only because that's when we often discover it! But in many cases it has had its beginning much earlier.

In a survey done in New Orleans, of several thousand people, about half the people found to have high blood pressure were over age fifty, and about half were younger.

One of the tragic aspects of high blood pressure is that it often strikes young and middle-aged adults—people in the prime of life, in their most productive years.

### Is a little high blood pressure normal in later years?

No. It used to be thought that blood pressure naturally rises with age, but now we know that this is by no means inevitable, and certainly not desirable.

Dr. William Harlan, of the University of Alabama Medical School, studied over one thousand pilots with the U.S. Naval Aerospace Medical Research Institute. The men were first studied at age twenty-four when they qualified for naval flight training and were followed for the next thirty years. Half the men had *no* rise in blood pressure at all in those thirty years.

And in Chicago, where Dr. Jeremiah Stamler and his team studied nine hundred men at the People's Gas, Light and Coke Company, they found that over a period of twenty years more than 30 percent of those men kept the same pressure as they had when younger.

And in both these studies, the men who did get high blood pressure were those who had pressures a little on the high side of normal when they were young. So let this be a warning sign: If you have pressure a little higher than normal when young, be sure to pay particular attention to it as you get older.

### Is it too late to treat in later years?

A person with high blood pressure is never too old to treat. Of course, the earlier you treat it, the better, because it hasn't had a chance to cause damage. Furthermore, the less severe the disease, the easier it is to treat. But no matter how long you have had the pressure, it is still important to have it treated.

### What about high blood pressure in children?

Some experts estimate that 1 to 2 percent of all children have high blood pressure. So play it safe and have your children's pressure checked regularly.

Pediatricians have not usually taken blood pressure as a routine procedure, but they are now being urged to do so. There is increasing evidence that high blood pressure, the kind stemming from unknown cause, is set up in childhood, the seeds planted, perhaps during the first two years of life, or even before birth. Blood pressure measurements should be a routine part of a child's physical examination.

One investigator in St. Louis found that thirty-two of forty children who had high blood pressure were overweight, which makes one think that obesity may be a factor in hypertension in childhood.

## *Does it occur in teen-agers?*

Yes. This aspect of the health watch over children should continue through the teen-age years. A study by the Health Research Council of the City of New York of students in several high schools showed a range of 2½ percent to 10 percent of students with elevated blood pressure.

Eight percent of high school students in inner city Washington were found to be hypertensive.

In Evans County, Georgia, 11 percent had high pressure. A University of Michigan survey of fourteen hundred college students showed about 20 percent had abnormally high pressure. And to show you how dangerous this condition can be in teen-agers, when thirty hypertensive teen-agers were traced after seven years, two had died of strokes, four had developed heart and brain symptoms.

There is increasing evidence that children and teen-agers whose blood pressure levels are in the upper range of the distribution curve are frequently those who will develop hypertension as adults even though at the time the measurements are made they are "normotensive" by adult standards.

Diastolic pressure of 85 in anyone under the age of eighteen usually indicates hypertension and should be treated.

One tragic condition called "berry aneurysm" seems to occur particularly in young girls who have moderately high blood pressure. It means that a tiny bubble forms on the side of a small artery, and when blood pressure becomes high, the bubble can suddenly burst, causing a stroke, or even death. It is not common, but the sudden death of a young person from this possible cause should be a reason for all relatives to have their blood pressure checked.

### Does high blood pressure run in families?

It certainly seems to. Doctors have observed clusters of high blood pressure patients in families, indicating that heredity plays a real role in the disease. If one your parents, or a brother or sister has high blood pressure, your chances of developing it are much higher than they would otherwise be.

Not that you should worry about that, but "it should raise your index of suspicion," says Dr. Campbell Moses of New York City, former medical director of the American Heart Association.

"You should be sure to tell your doctor about your parents' history of high blood pressure, so he can be alert to the possibility. And a parent with high blood pressure should tell his child's pediatrician so that he can be certain to make periodic checks. And if both your parents had high pressure, and yours is now a little high, you should really be discouraged from smoking and gaining weight."

Any time one person in the family has high blood pressure or dies at a young age from a stroke or heart disease, other members of the family should have checkups of their blood pressures at an early age, and should continue to have them checked every year.

In my own practice, I have several patients whose parents and siblings all died with a stroke or a heart attack before age fifty. A family history of hypertension is extremely important from two points of view: (1) It suggests essential rather than secondary hypertension, and (2) It may have important implications for a future prognosis. Platt has stated that a middle-aged brother or sister of a patient with severe hypertension has about eight times the chance of having high blood pressure as a person selected at random.

On the other side of the coin the age of the family member at the time of a hypertensive complication is important. Very often when a patient is asked whether a parent had high blood pressure, he says, "Oh yes! My mother did." Finding out that mother's age was eighty-five when she died and that her hypertension was discovered only two years before death is quite a different story from mother dying at age forty-two with a stroke.

Dr. Edward Kass of Harvard Medical School has found that a tendency toward high blood pressure can often be detected as early as age two in children whose parents have high pressure. The children, even at that age, have slightly higher than usual readings.

Dr. Kass and his colleagues believe that a kind of blood pressure "track" is established early in life, with the likelihood that people with higher than average pressures as children are candidates for more severe high blood pressure as adults.

A hereditary tendency to high blood pressure can occur in animals, too. Dr. Lewis K. Dahl, of Brookhaven National Laboratory in New York State, has been able to breed one strain of laboratory rats that develop hypertension easily.

### *If my mother or father had high blood pressure, will I get it?*

Not necessarily. You may get it, or you may not. However, you're more *likely* to get it than if your family inheritance is one of normal blood pressure. So you should check your pressure regularly to make sure it doesn't start going up without your knowing it.

## *Male and female*

High blood pressure occurs in both men and women. It seems to be more prevalent in men at early ages, but after that the rates even out. High pressure is less common in women than men before the age of menopause. But in the older ages, high blood pressure is more frequently found among women.

In women, heart disease, too, seems to run about ten years behind men. But there doesn't seem to be much difference between men and women in the occurrence of strokes or congestive heart failure.

However, men seem to have a more severe form of high blood pressure. Their death rate from the disease is significantly higher than in women.

## *Do women have a greater tolerance for high blood pressure?*

This is a common belief, but the greater mortality in men is almost wholly attributable to coronary attacks. So we might say that women tolerate hypertension better than men only as far as the heart aspect of the disease is concerned.

The amount of damage to the brain and kidneys from hypertension is the same in women as in men. And a woman is just as apt to get a stroke from high blood pressure as a man.

Heart attacks are still the leading cause of death in women as well as men.

As you can see, women are by no means immune to the damaging effects of hypertension. Man or woman, if your blood pressure is high, you should get it treated.

## Blacks and whites

High blood pressure claims far more victims among black people than white. In fact, high blood pressure is the biggest cause of death in blacks. For every black who dies of sickle cell anemia, one hundred die from hypertension.

About 15 percent of white adults and 28 percent of black adults have high blood pressure, according to most surveys. (Many recent surveys indicate that the percentages may be higher in both groups.)

Also, high blood pressure tends to come along earlier and to be more severe in blacks than whites.

Ten years ago, a National Health Examination Survey showed in people aged twenty-five to thirty-four about 3.7 percent of white men, but 12.5 percent of black men, had high blood pressure. For women in this same age group, it was 2.3 percent for whites, but 8.5 percent for blacks. And the disease causes more deaths in blacks.

In Kansas City, a recent study showed that the death rate from high blood pressure, and heart diseases associated with it, was ten times higher among non-whites between the ages of thirty-five and forty-four. And it was six times higher from those causes in the forty-five to seventy-four age group, says Dr. Samuel Rodgers, a black physician who heads the Wayne-Miner Community Health Center there.

"To be black and male, and with high blood pressure, makes you more likely to die," says Dr. Louis C. Brown, acting chairman of the Scientific Council of the National Medical Association.

Hypertension in blacks seems to be different somehow. Besides developing earlier in life, being frequently more severe, and resulting in a higher mortality at a young age, in blacks it causes more strokes. In whites, it causes more heart disease.

Our studies conducted in the Birth Control Clinic, D.C. General Hospital in Washington, have re-emphasized the high incidence of hypertension in young black women. A random sample of black patients attending the clinic showed 48 percent had a history of elevated blood pressure. The average age of the women was only twenty-three. Other studies conducted in the Toxemia Clinic at D.C. General Hospital showed that 70 percent of the patients originally diagnosed as having toxemia of pregnancy by the obstetricians actually had hypertensive vascular disease.

In Washington, 88 percent of the hypertensive deaths below the age of sixty were among blacks.

## What are the reasons for these black–white differences?

No one knows for sure. Heredity may play a role, as well as difference in life stresses and diet.

For example, what is the role of heavy salt in the diet? Most black people eat three to four times more salt than the average white person.

And what about the role of stress? No one would deny that the black man in most places has a much higher day-to-day stress rate than the white man.

## Where you live

High blood pressure is found in people everywhere.

City people are just as likely to get it as country people or suburbanites.

Hypertension has no geographical boundaries. In France, one out of every three men by the age of fifty has high blood pressure. In Africa, high blood pressure is said to account for more hospital admissions than all other cardiovascular diseases combined.

In fact, the problem is so worldwide that the World Health Organization is mounting a special crusade against it. Pilot studies to investigate how best to control it are being set up in several countries. And mass screening campaigns are, or are about to be, set up in a dozen or so countries.

However, there are some differences in susceptibility to high blood pressure according to where you live. In Peru, investigators find that people living high in the Andes have much lower pressures than their countrymen living at sea level. And if those who have high pressure living at sea level then move to higher attitude, their pressures gradually fall over several years.

In Japan, one group of people has an especially high rate of high blood pressure, the theory being that here it is not the geographical location, but the high salt exposure these people have working in the salt mines.

Medical opinion and findings differ on whether geography and factors associated with it have any bearing on development of high blood pressure. A few groups of people living in South Pacific islands and some tribes in Africa show little rise in blood pressure with age, but it still isn't clear whether this is associated with geography, the fact that they live in tropical climes, or whether it is due to heredity, diet, or a particular style of living. For example, these people usually do not gain weight with the passing years which may account for their greater freedom from high blood pressure and arterial disease.

One group of researchers believes some of the geographical differences might be due to trace elements in the soil and water. The concentration of cadmium in various places seems to be correlated with geographical differences in hypertension, according to the World Health Organization. And two studies on air pollution in U.S. cities show that the cadmium concentration in the air is correlated with heart disease, hypertension, and arteriosclerosis.

Some changes, such as the increase of nickel and manganese levels in patients with heart disease, are so sharp and rapid that they might be used as indicators for an early diagnosis of heart attack. Clinical and experimental studies indicate that chromium, zinc, manganese, and vanadium may exert beneficial effects on fat metabolism and atherosclerosis, whereas copper may increase atherosclerosis. Also, there is evidence that cardiovascular death rates are sometimes lower with hardness of drinking water. Areas served by hard water usually experience lower cardiovascular death rates than the areas served by soft water.

Some investigators report a high concentration of cadmium in the blood and kidneys of people with high blood pressure. Cadmium is known to cause high blood pressure on laboratory rats.

But all of the evidence against trace metals so far is fragmentary, and nothing consistent has been established.

The World Health Agency and the International Atomic Energy Agency are carrying out a joint research effort to analyze trace elements in various locations of the world and try to determine whether there is truly a relationship to high blood pressure and other cardiovascular diseases.

### *Do fat people get more high blood pressure than thin people?*

Obesity doesn't *cause* high blood pressure, but high blood pressure does occur more often in overweight people than in those who are of normal weight or on the thin side.

This was shown by the statistics gathered on people living in Framingham, Massachusetts, who were studied for more than twenty-five years in relation to heart and circulatory conditions. It was found that people with high blood pressure were on the average more overweight than people with normal pressure. And at all ages, the occurrence of high blood pressure increased with the relative weight.

The relationship of obesity to high blood pressure was also shown by a study done for over thirty years on pilots in naval flight training. The largest weight gains occurred at the same time as the largest increases in blood pressure, and the relationships continued throughout the entire thirty years.

Insurance figures also show that average blood pressure rises as body weight increases.

### *Do people who eat a lot of salt get more high blood pressure?*

Salt and high blood pressure have been thought for a long time to have a connection, but it is something that has been hard to prove one way or the other.

Dr. Lewis K. Dahl, of Brookhaven National Laboratories in New York, has been investigating salt and high blood pressure for some twenty years and believes firmly that there is a relationship. Some other doctors do not agree, and that's where it stands—not proved either way.

High quantities of salt have definitely been shown to cause high blood pressure in laboratory rats. And it has also been shown that if a human being eats very little salt, it will often lower high blood pressure. But is the reverse true: does it *cause* high blood pressure?

Dr. Dahl believes that excessive eating of salt triggers high blood pressure in those who already have an inherited tendency to develop the disease. This has been shown to be the mechanism in the rats he studied.

We also know that societies that have a higher average salt intake have a greater prevalence of high blood pressure than societies having a low average salt intake. For example, in one Japanese city, where people eat a phenomenally high thirty grams of salt per day, the rate of severe hypertension is very high.

### *What about exercise?*

Do people who sit on their rear ends all day have more high blood pressure than those who exercise regularly?

One study to determine this was done by Dr. Henry Montoye, of the University of Michigan. He investigated some sixteen hundred men and found that blood pressures were definitely lower in the more active man, and higher in the sedentary men.

Also, in England, postmen who walked from door to door had a lower incidence of heart disease than bus drivers who sat all day.

### *Do people under stress have more high blood pressure than others?*

Yes, a number of studies have shown this. But usually, stress is a temporary condition and so the effects of its raising pressure are also temporary.

For example, researchers have noted that the prevalence of high blood pressure went up as much as 300 percent during such stress times as a major earthquake or devastating fires. Studies of a number of men who were in danger of losing their jobs and then did lose them showed that their pressures were very high during the entire threatening time.

Other tests have shown that people's pressures rise when they are frustrated, or when insulting remarks are made to them.

One doctor who takes his blood pressure readings regularly found that his pressure shot up twenty-five points when he was separated for a time from the woman he loved.

But these are all short term situations. What we don't know is what the effects of long-term stress situations are, when people are caught up for years or a life time in situations over which they have no control.

Blacks living in middle-class suburbs in Detroit, for example, have lower blood pressures on the average than blacks living in the slums of the city. Is a difference in stress the reason? Or are there other changes in environment accounting for the difference?

### *Is there a personality type that tends to get high blood pressure?*

Contrary to what you might think, it is not the nervous, tense, uptight people only whose blood pressure is on the rise. You can be the coolest dude in town and still have high blood pressure. However, some investigators believe that a person may be more susceptible to high blood pressure if he feels or thinks more intensely than others, or if he experiences emotional upsets more often.

Several attempts have been made to pinpoint some kind of hypertensive personality. At the University of California, a group of women who had high blood pressure were studied over an eleven-year period for personality traits they might have in common. They appeared to share four characteristics: They tended to be hostile toward people, looking for hostility in others and often provoking it. They had an anxious, defensive attitude. They had failed to achieve roles in life appropriate to their age. And they tended to respond strongly to things.

In another study, of U.S. Air Force officers, those with high blood pressures, investigators said, were likely to be "dominant, assertive, decisive, task-oriented and tended to be leaders." Then as a second check, the investigators matched these men with other officers who had leadership qualities but had low blood pressure. The higher pressure men, they said, "tended to have narrow ranges of interest, low thresholds for perceiving threat, challenge and hostility in other people, and were over-controlling, rigid, stereotyped, and obtuse in their social relationships."

But other investigators point out that those groups

studied are small and not necessarily typical. Many people who do not have these characteristics also have high blood pressure. And many people who do seem uptight and defensive *don't* have high blood pressure.

The truth is that no convincing study has yet been done to prove that a particular personality type is associated with hypertension.

### Tie-ins with other conditions

Doctors are not sure why, but there seems to be a correlation between high blood pressure and glaucoma and between high blood pressure and diabetes.

People who have diabetes have a higher rate of high blood pressure than people who do not have diabetes. In fact, one-third to one-half of all diabetics have high blood pressure.

And two British ophthalmologists report that patients who have glaucoma with high tension of fluid inside the eyeball also tend to have higher blood pressure.

### The mosaic theory

Put it all together and what do you have? Some investigators say all of these things can be a major factor: that, actually, high blood pressure can be caused by many things; that a person may have an inherited tendency toward high blood pressure and then various factors may act on the tendency, and so trigger into a full-blown case of high pressure.

So, as you determine what groups of people—racially, hereditarily, or in terms of personality—you fall into, do not be alarmed if you seem to fit many of the groups at risk. The statistics don't mean you *will* get high blood pressure. They only mean the chances are a little higher that you *might* get high pressure. The more categories you fall into of people who especially tend to have high blood pressure, the higher the chances are that you might get it. As Dr. Moses has said, it should not scare you, but should "raise your index of suspicion."

The only way you can tell for sure is to have your blood pressure checked regularly.

# 4

## *What High Blood Pressure Is All About— The Inside Story*

Every time your heart beats, it pushes blood out into the circulatory system, putting it under pressure to move ahead. This is blood pressure—the pressure of your blood against the walls of your arteries and veins as it moves along.

Blood pressure is necessary to life. Without it, the blood could not circulate.

This pressure forces oxygen-laden blood to all parts of the body, driving it continuously throughout the thousands of miles of arteries and tiny capillaries and veins. Without pressure and circulation, your brain, heart, stomach, eyes, toes, liver, and other organs would soon hunger for oxygen, and would die.

So, the right level of blood pressure is good for you.

But *high* pressure can become a killer. It's like your automobile tires. Air pressure keeps your tires inflated. But over-inflation damages the tires, and makes the ride harder. It may even lead to a blowout. High blood pressure in a similar way over-inflates your arteries. Even a slight elevation can be harmful. (And, by the way, it takes longer to check the air pressure in your tires than to check your blood pressure.)

In this chapter we will look at what goes on in your body to keep your blood pressure at a normal level, and exactly what goes wrong to cause its elevation.

First, let's take a look at the normal circulatory system so that we can better understand the things that go wrong within it to produce circulatory problems and diseases.

## The heart

A chicken's heart looks just about the way your heart looks—dark red, shiny, a more or less solid mass of muscle. But your heart is bigger, about the size of your fist or a little larger.

If you close your fist hard and open it slowly, it gives you some idea of the action of your heart. This magnificent hunk of muscle that keeps your body alive contracts and relaxes this way some seventy times a minute, every minute of your life. This adds up to some one hundred thousand times a day, almost forty million times a year. And all without a rest.

There are four hollow chambers inside the heart: the two at the top are called atria, and the two at the bottom are called ventricles. They are separated by walls of muscle. When the heart relaxes, some blood comes into the top right atrium from the body, and other blood comes into the left atrium from the lungs. The two atria contract, squeezing the blood down into the ventricles. Then the ventricles contract, shooting the blood out; one ventricle sending the blood through the main artery to the body, and the other one sending the blood through the pulmonary artery to the lungs.

Inside the heart are valves that slap shut when the heart contracts, keeping the blood going in the right direction without backing up. The slapping shut of these valves is what makes the sound of your heart beat.

## *The pulse*

When the heart contracts, the blood surges out with a great deal of pressure behind it. As this pressure hits the blood in the arteries it is carried along, so you feel the beat of your pulse with every beat of the heart, normally seventy-two beats per minute, higher with exercise or excitement.

## *Your blood vessels*

Between the tiny branches of arteries and veins that go throughout the body are even smaller arterioles and then the very tiniest of blood vessels, called the capillaries. It is the capillaries that carry the blood to the individual cells of all the organs of the body where oxygen and other chemicals are delivered and carbon dioxide and other waste products are collected. The capillaries then connect with small veins which run into larger veins and thus back to the heart.

The sum total of this network of arteries, veins and capillaries forms some seventy thousand miles of passageway for the blood to flow through.

Blood flow is very slow in the capillaries. It takes an entire minute for the blood to go through just one inch of a capillary vessel. In contrast, the blood roars through the major arteries at a speed of more than forty miles an hour! The slow trip through the capillaries is required so that food, chemicals, and oxygen needed by the body cells can pass through the walls of the tiny capillaries and into the tissue. In the same way, used carbon dioxide and other waste products enter the capillaries to be carried away.

You can get an idea of how fine an operation this whole capillary action is if you picture the red blood cells as being so small that if you stacked three thousand of them in line it wouldn't even make one inch. Or, you could hide forty or fifty of them together at the end of this sentence, under the period. In turn, the capillaries are so small that these red blood cells have to squeeze through them in single file.

## *The pressure*

If we follow along the arteries as they branch into smaller and smaller channels, like the branches of a tree, we come to the tiny arterioles, skinnier than the tiniest hairs. It is here that blood pressure is controlled. All over the body these arterioles contract or expand to control the flow of blood into various parts of the body. When they contract in one part of the body, it makes it harder for the blood to flow through there. It's like a nozzle regulating the water pressure in a garden hose. Make the nozzle opening narrower, and the water comes out under more pressure. When the arterioles clamp down, the blood backs up in the larger arteries, and blood pressure increases.

Part of this process is normal. Its function is used to shoot blood from one part of the body to another as it's needed. If a two-headed, three-horned monster should start chasing you down the street, you want your legs to move! So the arterioles in your stomach clamp down, the arterioles in your legs open up, and your leg muscles get the energy-giving blood so they can do their job.

But when the arterioles are constantly clamped down, wholesale, all over the body, it makes the blood pressure go up and stay up, and that's bad.

In addition to the arterioles, there are two other factors that are important in determining what your blood pressure is. One is the output of the heart—just how much blood it is pumping into the system. The amount can vary tremendously, depending on whether you are resting or are exercising strenuously.

The circulatory system is a closed system, remember, so your pressure depends on how much blood is being pumped in and how much resistance there is to it. What goes in depends on the heart and how much it pumps. How much resistance there is depends partly on how tight or relaxed your arterioles are, but it also depends a great deal on that other factor mentioned previously—your kidneys. At least one fourth of the total output of blood from the heart goes to the kidneys. If there is a problem with the circulation of the kidneys, as there often is in high blood pressure, then the resistance to the flow of blood is greatly increased, thus raising pressure.

### *The super-controllers*

What controls the arterioles and the heart and the kidneys that in turn control the blood pressure?

Actually, there is a whole system of controls. These controllers send the signals out to change your blood pressure as your needs change, decreasing it when you sleep, increasing it enough when you stand up so your blood can make the uphill climb to reach your brain, increasing it even more when you have to run or work hard or are afraid.

One of the super-controllers is a group of cells in the arteries going up your neck (the carotid arteries). These cells are sensitive to changes in pressure of the blood around them. As the thermostat is set for a certain temperature on a furnace, these cells, called baroreceptors, are tuned to a certain narrow range of blood pressure. When the pressure goes above or below that range, they send signals to a center in the base of the brain to increase or decrease the pressure as needed.

Actually there are a number of these pressure-receptors all over the body in various important arteries, but the one in the neck is the most important one. You can check it by pressing hard on the sides of your neck near the base. As you increase the pressure on your neck, your blood pressure will fall, and you'll quickly feel dizzy.

The other super-controller is the nervous system. One of your nervous systems—you've got several—is the sympathetic system. It sends signals out to increase the heart rate, constrict blood vessels, and raise blood pressure. The other nervous system is the parasympathetic system. It acts to lower the heart rate, relax the blood vessels, and lower blood pressure. These two systems act in a set of checks and balances to produce the proper blood pressure, depending on your needs at any one moment.

In addition to these super-controllers, we have the action of hormones. The adrenal glands, for example, secrete two hormones that are powerful increasers of blood pressure. They manufacture hormones in great quantities during exercise or during emotional stress. The kidney manufactures the hormone renin that also raises pressure. There are also other hormones and chemicals circulating in the blood that can modify what these super-controllers dictate by increasing or decreasing the effects of the command signals.

It's a fantastically complex system in which all these factors can operate alone and also interact with each other.

It is so complex that researchers had to put the entire system into a computer to try to analyze the various effects on the blood pressure when any one or two of the factors involved are changed.

## Why is blood pressure expressed in two numbers, like 130/85?

Because you have two kinds of blood pressure.

One is the systolic pressure, when your heart is contracting and pumping out blood. The other is the diastolic pressure, when your heart is resting between beats, that is, it's the minimum pressure that is constantly present in your arteries. A blood pressure of 130/85 means a systolic or beating pressure of 130, and a diastolic or constant pressure of 85. (The numbers refer to millimeters of mercury—how

far a tiny column of mercury is forced up a pressure-meas-
uring scale.)

## What's the desirable reading?

The lower the reading the better. A study by life insurance
companies shows that the higher a person's blood pressure
rises, the shorter his life expectancy.

We'll show you in the next chapter exactly how to figure
your own life expectancy based on your age, sex, and blood
pressure.

## Do doctors agree upon a desirable pressure?

No, because there is no one best pressure for everyone. Age
makes a difference. So do sex and other factors. The range
for normal systolic pressure can be anywhere between 100
and 140. Normal diastolic pressure is anywhere from 60 to
90. In general, 120/80 is considered an average good
pressure. All the medical evidence points to a longer,
healthier life the lower you can keep your pressure.

## Can your pressure ever be too low?

Unless very low blood pressure is associated with some
disease or causes you to be dizzy, it is nothing to worry
about. The lower the better. As Dr. William Kannel of the
National Heart and Lung Institute says, "An ideal blood
pressure would be the lowest pressure you could achieve
without going into shock."

## *What do the doctors consider high blood pressure?*

The World Health Organization considers 140/90 and below as normal, and 160/95 and over as hypertensive. Anything in between is considered borderline. Actually, there is a gradual curve of blood pressures from low to very high, the line between "normal" and "high" being an arbitrary line. To define *high* is like trying to define how high is up. In addition, each person's blood pressure fluctuates from hour to hour, and can change within seconds.

Dr. Theodore Cooper, director of the National Heart and Lung Institute and chairman of the government's interagency commission against high blood pressure, talks about it this way: "Almost with no limit, the higher your blood pressure is, the more you're at risk. Now, for insurance purposes and for many other reasons of practicality, we have tended to settle on a diastolic pressure of 90 or 95 as being a level at which there is some reason to become alarmed or to think of doing something.

"Whether you choose 90 or 95 isn't too important. First of all, we don't measure blood pressure this accurately and to think that we're really drawing a meaningful distinction between 90 and 95 is illusory. When the patient isn't at rest, 95 may be a reasonable level. If one has the patient more at rest, and if he has been seen several times, perhaps 90 is a more meaningful value. Blood pressure tends to be higher when a person is in a strained situation where he is alarmed or doesn't know the physician, or where there are other people looking on."

The following classifications for blood pressure are generally accepted by medical authorities:

NORMAL PRESSURE:
    Systolic (upper number) pressure of 100–140
    Diastolic (lower number) pressure of 60–90

BORDERLINE OR MILD HYPERTENSION:
  Systolic pressure of 140–160
  Diastolic pressure of 90–95
MODERATE HYPERTENSION:
  Systolic pressure of 160–180
  Diastolic pressure of 96–114
MARKED HYPERTENSION:
  Systolic pressure above 180
  Diastolic pressure above 115

### *Everybody talks about diastolic pressure: isn't systolic important?*

They are both important. There is the same kind of organ damage and early death rate from high systolic pressure as there is from high diastolic pressure. It's just that most of the research has been done on diastolic pressure.

Actually, when one goes up, the other usually goes up too.

Some doctors like to come to decisions by adding the diastolic pressure and systolic pressure together. If the sum is 250 or higher, treatment needs to be obtained promptly. In some clinics, the assistant under these circumstances is instructed to leave the room to contact a physician immediately to make sure that the person does not leave before receiving additional evaluation and starting treatment.

### *What is hypertension?*

That's another name for high blood pressure. Many people think hypertension means general tenseness and anxiety. This is not true. Hypertension does NOT mean being tense and nervous. It simply means excessive blood pressure in your arteries. It means hyper (high) tension (pressure) of blood within arteries.

You can be very angry or very tense over something and yet *not* have high blood pressure. Emotions and stress *can* play a role in causing high blood pressure, but they don't *necessarily* go together.

### What is meant by "essential hypertension?"

"Essential" does *not* mean "necessary." "Essential hypertension" simply means high blood pressure of unknown cause, which is true in most cases. You may also hear the term "benign" hypertension. Benign means mild, harmless. But the term is rarely used now, since there is never anything harmless about high blood pressure.

### Can the risk of harm from a given degree of elevated pressure vary with individuals?

Yes. Occasionally, you may hear of someone who had an astonishingly high pressure but lived to be eighty-five years old. But such individuals are extremely rare.

### Does blood pressure rise with age?

Usually, but not always. It's not an automatic part of growing older. It used to be thought that your blood pressure was okay if it was 100 plus your age. Now studies show that this is not true. Now we know that even a slight rise in pressure can be dangerous.

### Is your blood pressure always the same?

No. As we said earlier it can vary from day to day, even hour by hour or minute by minute. It is raised by anger, fear, pain, and cold, and also goes up when you are excited, engaged in strenuous exercise, or under emotional stress. It goes down when you are resting, relaxed, watching television, or sleeping; in fact, it may drop to half the level during sleep as when awake. These variations can apply to the diastolic pressure as well as the systolic.

Sometimes during sleep, pressure drops to levels as surprisingly low as 60/40.

Blood pressure not only varies greatly from moment to moment, but it also has a regular daily rhythm, being lowest in the morning when you wake up and then increasing during the day until the early evening hours, when it begins to drop again.

These variations have been discovered by having people wear portable blood pressure devices all day long, with pressure automatically recorded moment by moment.

Sir George Pickering, the noted British cardiologist, showed slides at a medical meeting of such recordings. One slide reported the arterial pressure changes in a volunteer subject over a twenty-four-hour period: during sleep, walking, on receiving an injection—which caused it to rise—and finally when making love to his wife. (During intercourse, diastolic pressure of normal subjects has been found to rise some 30 to 40 points.)

Commenting on this last action, Sir George said: "You can see that the arterial pressure rises quite high. . . . And then afterwards he falls asleep." When this was shown to the physiological society at Oxford, one scientist, a redheaded Greek lady, said, "Just like a bloody Britisher! Turns over and goes to sleep."

Dr. Pickering tells another story of an automatic device hooked up to one of the doctors as he went on hospital rounds with Dr. Pickering.

"Dr. Bevan was standing listening to me conducting a ward round. His arterial pressure was surprisingly low, at a level of 80/50. He was clearly bored, perhaps almost asleep," says Dr. Pickering.

But he adds, "The head nurse stuck a pin into his behind, and his pressure rose abruptly to 150/70!"

## Has research been able to show what causes high blood pressure?

No. While it explains what happens to cause high blood pressure for short periods, it still doesn't explain what happens to cause day-in-day-out high blood pressure, the kind that pounds at your arteries and causes so much damage.

As one well-known cardiologist said: "What causes hypertension? We don't have the foggiest notion."

## What are the theories concerning the underlying causes of high blood pressure?

1. There is some evidence that it may be due to a goof-up in body chemistry, that your kidneys or adrenal glands put out some hormones or other chemicals that cause blood pressure to go up.

2. A super-sensitive nervous system might over-react to stress and cause the arterioles to close down.

3. High blood pressure tends to run in families, so heredity apparently plays some role. If your parents have high blood pressure, your chances of developing it are much greater.

4. A number of doctors think that the high salt content in our food from infancy on could be a cause or at least a contributory factor.

5. Some evidence is turning up that tiny amounts of certain metals and chemicals in the water supply, such as cadmium, can cause high blood pressure.

Each of the above theories has some evidence going for it, but each is still controversial.

## *What makes some people get high blood pressure, but not others?*

That's another missing link in present knowledge. There may be many reasons. A person may have a genetic predisposition for high blood pressure, and various things could actually trigger off the rise. In 90 percent of cases, we simply don't know the cause, and we call the problem "essential hypertension."

## *What about the 10 percent of high blood pressure with known causes?*

Certain kidney diseases are known to cause hypertension, or obstructions to the arteries leading to one kidney can restrict blood flow or cause the kidney to release chemicals that raise blood pressure. Sometimes the kidney arteries become plugged up with fatty deposits, or one muscle around these arteries constricts them.

A tumor of the adrenal gland is also a known cause. The tumor secretes extra amounts of a hormone that in turn affects the kidneys; salt and water are not excreted properly, and high blood pressure results. When the tumor is removed by surgery, the high pressure is usually cured.

Sometimes high blood pressure is caused by a malformation of the aorta, the main artery coming from the heart. It can also be corrected by surgery.

We'll talk about these more rare forms of high blood pressure in a later chapter.

### *What about high blood pressure in pregnancy?*

High blood pressure frequently occurs in pregnancy, even when the woman had normal pressure before becoming pregnant. On the other hand, mysteriously, sometimes a hypertensive woman prior to pregnancy may become normotensive during pregnancy.

High blood pressure is sometimes a warning of a condition called toxemia of pregnancy. In toxemia, in addition to the high blood pressure, there is retention of fluid in the tissues, which causes swollen legs and feet, as well as damage to the kidneys. This is dangerous for both mother and unborn baby, and calls for immediate treatment.

# 5

## Why High Blood Pressure Is Dangerous

Every year 2.5 million Americans are hit during their daily activities or silently in the middle of the night by stroke. Some recover, others are crippled, perhaps unable to walk or talk for the rest of their lives.

Every year ambulances scream through the streets, rushing to the hospital more than one million Americans overcome by heart attacks. Nearly seven hundred thousand of them die, some without ever reaching the hospital.

Every year tens of thousands develop heart failure, and die of it.

Every year thousands of others die of kidney failure, the poisons slowly building up in their bodies until the body can no longer survive.

And the numbers are multiplied in other countries throughout the world. That is why high blood pressure is so dangerous. It is a leading factor, sometimes the only one, in the causes of all these deaths. It is certainly the commonest cause of all deaths in blacks. In fact, some medical scientists consider it the leading factor in the total number of deaths from all causes in people throughout the world.

In addition, high blood pressure can cause blindness. It is

a major factor in increasing fatty deposits in atherosclerosis. It is a major factor in arteriosclerosis (hardening of the arteries), and may well be a major reason for the loss of memory and brain breakdown in old age.

Aside from the people it kills, there are millions who are robbed of their natural health and strength by high blood pressure. Undiagnosed and untreated, they are unable to enjoy their lives completely, to do the everyday things that most of us take for granted.

You may feel and look young and healthy, at the prime of your life. But how old are your blood vessels right now? Are they healthy, too, or are they—hidden from your view—old before their time?

Only your doctor—and your blood pressure number—can tell you.

### How does high blood pressure cause damage?

By putting extra damaging pressure on your blood vessels with every beat of the heart! Not only does this damage the blood vessels in a direct, physical way, but research indicates that it also causes a speed-up in arteriosclerosis (hardening of the arteries) and an increase in atherosclerosis (the laying down of fatty deposits inside arteries that can cause heart attack and strokes).

One researcher inserted tiny plexiglass windows in the skulls of rats to watch high blood pressure at work, and actually saw arteries in the rats' brains going into spasm and closing down.

Pounding high blood pressure over the years can also cause thickening of the walls of the blood vessels and progressive narrowing of the passageway. The prolonged stretching of the walls fragments the elastic fibers. The walls can become soft and give way, or they can become hardened, less elastic, scarred, and brittle.

Some of this occurs naturally with age. But high blood

pressure speeds up the process drastically. Soon the blood vessels can't deliver the necessary blood supply to vital organs. Or hemorrhage may occur through the damaged walls. Or a clot from the thickened walls may break off and go to the brain or heart.

Or sometimes a weakened wall will protrude like a thin-skinned balloon, in what is called an aneurysm. These can be tiny microscopic aneurysms in the brain or huge football-sized aneurysms of the main aorta. They are truly time bombs ready to burst in a second with any severe increase in blood pressure.

### What are the major organs that are damaged?

In addition to the blood vessels themselves, the main target organs that we know about are the heart, the kidneys, and the brain. But other organs can be affected by the pounding high pressures, too. For example, the eyes are affected in many people, and if high pressure is ignored for a long time, it can cause difficulties in vision, or even blindness.

Remember the probable president of the AMA who had untreated high blood pressure for twenty-five years and then died of it? His pathology report at autopsy showed how terribly widespread blood pressure damage can be. Severe hardening and narrowing of the arteries in the heart, kidney, and brain. Holes in brain cells, and severe degeneration. Enlarged heart fibers. Scarring. Blood vessels in the heart 50 percent blocked by narrowing. Kidney tissue hardened. Hardening of the kidney blood vessels. Liver congested. Death of many liver cells. Spleen and adrenal glands congested and swollen. Lungs congested, and inflamed.

All this could have been prevented.

### What does high blood pressure specifically do to your heart and circulation?

High blood pressure is primarily a disease of blood vessels. The first abnormality is a narrowing of the smallest blood vessels (arterioles) which take the blood from the heart. A good analogy is to think of the blood vessels as your pipes and your heart as the pump. Once the small blood vessels become narrow, your heart (the pump), which is a group of muscles similar to any other muscles in your body, is forced to work harder to pump the blood through the narrow pipes.

Just as the muscle in your arm enlarges when you dig a ditch or work in your garden, so your heart muscle enlarges when it is forced to work harder to push the blood through narrowed arteries.

### Congestive heart failure

The heart muscle can enlarge only so far before its fibers begin to stretch, which makes its pumping action ineffectual. Each contraction of the heart pump from that time on fails to empty its contents entirely, causing a backup of blood into the blood vessels of the lungs and a sluggish circulation all over the body. As the heart pump becomes more ineffectual, it has a harder time pumping the blood around your body. Its poor pumping action fails to get all the blood back from your feet and legs and it begins to accumulate there with the result that you get swollen ankles or what the Bible refers to as "dropsy." In proportion to the failure of the heart pump, the fluid begins to accumulate in the tissues closer to the heart—in the thighs, abdomen, and lungs, and finally throughout the body.

Other symptoms are fatigue and shortness of breath, first on exertion and, finally, even at rest.

What we have been describing is called congestive heart failure or enlargement of the heart, which is a direct result of elevated blood pressure.

Once congestive heart failure develops, it can be very serious. It should be emphasized, however, that controlling the blood pressure *prevents* the development of congestive heart failure, giving a much better prognosis. Congestive heart failure is an absolutely preventable complication of high blood pressure. With early application of modern-day therapy, the hypertensive should *never* die because of this complication.

For example, Mrs. D.C., aged forty-nine, came into my office one day complaining of shortness of breath after climbing two flights of stairs, a fair amount of fatigue, and swelling of the ankles, particularly at the end of the day. All these symptoms had gradually gotten worse over the previous six months. Her blood pressure was first discovered to be high when she was going through the menopause some five years earlier. No therapy was given at that time.

Physical examination revealed her blood pressure to be 150/100 mm Hg. The blood vessels in the back of her eyes revealed signs of arteriosclerosis. Her heart was enlarged. The bottom of both her lungs contained a fair amount of fluid and there was swelling of her ankles and legs halfway up to her knees.

Digitalis, a medication that helps the heart perform more efficiently, was administered as well as a diuretic to get rid of the fluid. In a week's time Mrs. D.C. had lost eight pounds, the swelling was gone and, remarkably enough, her blood pressure was now 120/80 mm Hg. Frequently the clearing of heart failure brings the blood pressure down to normal. However, if antihypertensive medications had been given when her blood pressure was first discovered to be high, her heart would never have failed.

## *Angina*

High blood pressure significantly speeds up hardening of the arteries, especially of the arteries supplying the heart, the brain, and the kidneys. When the coronary arteries become involved, there may be a decrease in the blood supply to a particular part of the heart muscle. When this occurs, there is a squeezing-type pain (never sharp) in the middle of the chest (under the breastbone, not over the heart). This characteristic pain is known as "angina" and is caused by spasm of the muscle crying out for oxygen.

A.R., a fifty-three-year-old executive, for five years had suffered from hypertension which unfortunately had never been treated. He complained of pain under his breastbone which radiated up to his jaw and down his left arm when he walked uphill, particularly in cold weather or when he lifted anything.

Physical examination revealed a blood pressure of 150/100 mm Hg. The blood vessels in back of his eyes showed arteriosclerosis. His heart was not enlarged. The lungs were clear and there was no swelling of the ankles.

An electrocardiogram showed signs of hardening of the coronary arteries without any enlargement of the heart. He was instructed to put a tablet of nitroglycerin under his tongue before he either exerted himself or lifted anything and was placed on a thiazide diuretic for his blood pressure.

In two weeks time the chest pain had significantly decreased to the point that he required only three nitroglycerin tablets a day. His blood pressure was now 140/100 mm Hg. I therefore added reserpine to the thiazide diuretic.

When seen three weeks later the chest pain had entirely disappeared so that he now could lead a normal life without nitroglycerin. Controlling the blood pressure in this patient significantly improved his angina.

## *Heart attacks*

A lack of oxygen can also make the heart muscle irritable, causing it to beat irregularly—either too slow or too fast. This irritability of the heart muscle is the commonest cause of death if the heart survives the initial shock. Constant monitoring of the heart, and prompt use of drugs to regulate its rhythm, as is done routinely in intensive care units, have greatly decreased this complication and significantly decreased the number of deaths from heart attack. It is still much easier to prevent heart attacks in the first place, and controlling blood pressure certainly helps.

If there is complete blockage of blood supply to one area of the heart, either because of narrowing of the artery or because of a clot lodging there, then no nutrition or oxygen can get to that area of muscle. This results in tissue death which is known as a coronary infarction (a heart attack).

The degree of tissue death depends upon the size of the plugged artery and on whether the plugging took place all at once or gradually. If the involved artery is large, and the plug occurred rapidly, there is a large amount of tissue death, and sudden death is the usual result. (Heart attack is the commonest cause of sudden death).

If a smaller branch is involved and the plugging is either gradual or sudden, the seriousness depends on how well the heart muscle can withstand the insult.

There are many unanswered questions about heart attacks and high blood pressure. There is a definite tie-in, statistics show, but the tie-in is not as strong as the link between high blood pressure and congestive heart failure.

## *Brain damage*

High blood pressure can cause damage to the brain in several ways.

It can cause gradual damage by narrowing the arteries to a particular part of the brain, or by partially clogging them so that they do not deliver enough blood to that area. Spells of dizziness and confusion are often the symptoms when this occurs.

It can cause increased atherosclerosis and arteriosclerosis, with gradual deterioration of brain function.

A clot can form in an artery, cutting off circulation entirely and causing a stroke, just as a clot in the heart cuts off circulation and causes a heart attack.

Or a stroke may be caused by a blowout of an artery. High pressure over the years so weakens an artery wall that one final surge of pressure causes the weakened wall to burst, causing hemorrhage and brain damage.

High pressure can also cause swelling of the brain tissue, called hypertensive encephalopathy. This is an emergency situation producing violent headache, convulsions, coma, and sometimes death.

### Are heart attacks and strokes always caused by high blood pressure?

No, people with normal pressure can also be victims of these because of other causes that damage arteries or make blood clots form.

But the person with high pressure is much more likely to have a heart attack or stroke than the one with normal pressure.

### What makes one person with high blood pressure get a heart attack or stroke, and not another?

We do not know why. Apparently, different people have different abilities to tolerate high blood pressure.

But because there are these individual differences, it is

important to keep in close touch with your doctor so that he can check on you as an individual.

## Kidney damage

As the arteries become clogged up and circulation decreases, the kidneys do not get enough blood. They no longer function at full capacity in getting rid of body waste products from your blood. Salt is retained and fluid is retained because of the salt. You have to urinate more, particularly at night. (The kidneys work more efficiently when you are lying down and use the time when you are sleeping to rid the body of its waste products.)

The extra fluid puts more burden on the heart, creating a vicious cycle. As kidney tissue becomes destroyed, function gets worse and worse, uremic poisoning may occur, and even death.

## The problem of water build-up

One of the consequences of both congestive heart failure and damage to the kidneys is the build-up of water in the tissues. Our circulatory system and our body tissues are intricately balanced as to the amounts of fluids and the concentration of minerals and other chemicals they contain. We take in fluid with our food and drink. We give out fluid in urine, breathing and sweating. All of this is in delicate balance; if anything makes us get rid of less fluid, such as an inefficient heart or damaged kidneys, then the tissues become waterlogged, a condition called edema.

## Hypertension and atherosclerosis

There is no question that hypertension speeds up atherosclerosis, the process of corrosion of our arteries that so commonly leads to heart attack and stroke. And the higher the blood pressure, the faster this damaging process proceeds.

The effect of high blood pressure on atherosclerosis is seldom heard about, and yet it may be one of the significant ways in which high blood pressure causes damage.

Striking evidence turns up in such studies as one on arteries at 500 autopsies, done by Dr. Campbell Moses at the University of Pittsburgh before he became medical director of the American Heart Association. Dr. Moses found a marked increase in the frequency and severity of atherosclerosis in the hearts and brains of men and women who had high blood pressure as compared to those with normal pressures.

Apparently, high blood pressure is what turns a cholesterol-rich diet into a dangerous one. Animals fed a diet heavy with cholesterol will not have atherosclerosis if they have normal blood pressure.

With high blood pressure, that same diet—or even one lower in cholesterol—caused severe atherosclerosis in the animals, and often led to heart attacks. A high cholesterol diet had an adverse effect *only* if the animal had high blood pressure. There are tremendous implications here for human beings trying to avoid heart troubles.

This same process of high blood pressure increasing hardening of the arteries may also play a role when it comes to the forgetfulness and other brain deterioration of old age.

Some evidence for this was shown by studies done by Dr. Carl Eisdorfer at Duke University's Center for the Study of Aging. He and his associates observed 200 men and women in their sixties and seventies over a ten-year period. During that time, blood pressures were taken, and each patient regularly received a battery of intelligence tests.

Patients who had normal blood pressures showed almost no intellectual changes at the end of ten years; those with high blood pressure dropped almost ten points in test scores.

## *Eye damage*

How much damage does hypertension do to the eyes? A great deal.

The ophthalmoscope (that instrument we use to look at the back of your eyes) enables the doctor to see your blood vessels as they can be seen in no other part of the body. The whole process of how the elevated blood pressure worsens the arteriosclerotic process can be seen through this instrument.

Sam R. was a patient who wouldn't take his pills. With the ophthalmoscope, we could actually see his arteries getting worse. With mild high blood pressure, we could see the arteries begin to narrow until, as the severity of the disease increased, they became so narrow that we could hardly see them. Just as it must have been doing in the brain and kidneys, this narrowing reached a point where there was insufficient blood supply going to the capillaries with resultant tissue death. Every time we examined Sam, we could see deterioration of blood vessels, finally with production of hemorrhages and blindness.

One ophthalmologist, Dr. Donald Tucker, wrote in the Journal of the American Medical Association:

"Each year I see patients partially blinded by complications of hypertension. Most of these patients have had periodic physical examinations, but prior to their visual insult received no therapy or work-up for previously recognized hypertension."

In his practice, he said, more patients were blinded as a consequence of high blood pressure than by glaucoma, a well-known cause of blindness.

## Will taking hypertension drugs decrease risk of these damages?

Yes. The primary purpose of taking the medicines to reduce high blood pressure is to avoid the risk of target organ damage.

You may feel all right now, but it could hurt later as these organs deteriorate. And taking the medicine can prevent the damage that hurts.

Even if some damage has already occurred, taking the medicines can still help. People with high blood pressure who have had a stroke, for example, have less chance of having a second stroke if they take medicine to lower their blood pressure.

One of the problems is that people don't realize how dangerous high blood pressure is and just what it can do. A survey by Louis Harris and Associates showed that people with high blood pressure between the ages of seventeen and thirty-five, often don't regard high pressure as very serious. Yet these are the ones who are most in danger.

The need for education, so that people will obtain screening and treatment, is imperative. Such a program has only just begun. Where you can go for such screening and treatment will be discussed in the next chapter.

But, first, let us look at the results of some of the population studies that show more clearly than anything else the dangers of high blood pressure.

## The evidence

There are a number of important studies that have been done that show these dangers very dramatically (perhaps a better word would be *tragically*). Insurance statistics tell the most.

The largest sets of statistics come from a study, well known to physicians and insurance experts, called the Build and Blood Pressure Study. It includes statistics from twenty-six large life insurance companies and covers some 4 million men and women policy holders.

This study showed that people with blood pressure higher than 140/90 mm Hg., if it is untreated, die at an earlier age than people who have a lower pressure. The higher the blood pressure, the more years of life lost.

In fact, even blood pressure only slightly higher than 140/90 can mean a loss of years of life. In the study, for example, a man over age forty with a pressure of 150/100 had a mortality rate of 225 percent over the standard risk person.

A man with a pressure as high as 178/108 showed a mortality rate of about 600 percent!

Even within the normal range, those with lower pressures lived longer than those with higher normals.

### Life expectancy and elevated blood pressure

From the statistics of the Build and Blood Pressure Study, a person can determine what his life expectancy is at any given age and any given blood pressure.

For example, in the following tables you can see that, everything else being equal, if you are a man aged thirty-five, with a normal blood pressure, you can expect to live to be seventy-six and a half years old. However, if your blood pressure at age thirty-five is 150/100, you can only expect to live to be sixty, a loss of sixteen and a half years.

All of these statistics are for persons with high blood pressure that is untreated. If you lower your blood pressure with proper treatment, the picture is entirely different.

You can see from these statistics that, to a large extent, your blood pressure tells how long and how well you will live.

## MEN

### AGE 35

| Blood Pressure | Expected Age | Loss in Life Expectancy |
|---|---|---|
| Normal | $76\frac{1}{2}$ | — |
| 130/90 | $72\frac{1}{2}$ | 4 |
| 140/95 | $67\frac{1}{2}$ | 9 |
| 150/100 | 60 | $16\frac{1}{2}$ |

### AGE 45

| Blood Pressure | Expected Age | Loss in Life Expectancy |
|---|---|---|
| Normal | 77 | — |
| 130/90 | 74 | 3 |
| 140/95 | 71 | 6 |
| 150/100 | 60 | $11\frac{1}{2}$ |

### AGE 55

| Blood Pressure | Expected Age | Loss in Life Expectancy |
|---|---|---|
| Normal | $78\frac{1}{2}$ | — |
| 130/90 | $77\frac{1}{2}$ | 1 |
| 140/95 | $74\frac{1}{2}$ | 4 |
| 150/100 | $72\frac{1}{2}$ | 6 |

## WOMEN

### AGE 45

| Blood Pressure | Expected Age | Loss in Life Expectancy |
|---|---|---|
| Normal | 82 | — |
| 130/90 | $80\frac{1}{2}$ | $1\frac{1}{2}$ |
| 140/95 | 77 | 5 |
| 150/100 | $73\frac{1}{2}$ | $8\frac{1}{2}$ |

### AGE 55

| Blood Pressure | Expected Age | Loss in Life Expectancy |
|---|---|---|
| Normal | $82\frac{1}{2}$ | — |
| 130/90 | 82 | $\frac{1}{2}$ |
| 140/95 | $79\frac{1}{2}$ | 3 |
| 150/100 | $78\frac{1}{2}$ | 4 |

## The Framingham study

Framingham, Massachusetts, has been for years a living laboratory, where more than five thousand men and women living there, about twenty miles from Boston, have been studied in great detail. The entire town became an experiment. Physicians and statisticians and various members of their investigative teams have examined, probed, questioned, and studied the members of this community for nearly twenty-five years now. The goal—to learn more about heart disease and stroke, to learn how different factors affect them, and to learn whether differences in lifestyle can help prevent them.

The investigators have studied everything from inadequate sleep to coffee use to determine if they had any effect on the risk of getting a heart attack or stroke. As they kept track over the years, they found that the risk was greatly increased by smoking, by elevated levels of cholesterol, by lack of exercise, or by being overweight. But the prime factor they found in increasing the risk of stroke and heart attack was high blood pressure.

Over a fourteen-year period, heart attacks were three to five times more common in people who had hypertension than in those who did not. And the risk of stroke was four times higher in persons with high blood pressure than in those without.

Congestive heart failure was five times greater among the persons with high blood pressure as among those with normal pressure.

Dr. William B. Kannel urges persons with high blood pressure, no matter how old, to obtain treatment. "To await the onset of symptoms in hypertensive elderly persons before implementing therapy," he says, "is to invite the occurrence of a stroke."

Said Dr. Thomas R. Dawber, medical director of the

study, "If we could keep blood pressure down, it would do more good than anything else."

## The Chicago study

More evidence was piled on in a study begun in 1958 in Chicago, where Dr. Jeremiah Stamler, now with Northwestern University Medical School, investigated sixteen hundred men in their forties and fifties who worked at the People's Gas Company. When the men were followed closely for ten years, Dr. Stamler and his team of investigators found without any question the death rate during the ten years was precisely related to the men's blood pressure. Of men with normal blood pressure of 80 diastolic, only eight out of one hundred died in the ten years from all causes. Of men with high pressure, over 110 diastolic, thirty-seven out of every one hundred died.

And the same results were found as in the insurance and Framingham studies: that even the men with only mildly high pressures had a higher risk of death. Men with *mildly* raised pressures of only 90 to 99 diastolic had twice the death rate from all causes during the ten years as the men with a pressure of 80. And when you got down to deaths caused by cardiovascular diseases alone, the figures were even more tragic. In the men with mild high blood pressure compared with the men of normal pressures:

1. their risk of fatal cardiovascular-renal diseases was doubled;

2. their risk of coronary disease was trebled;

3. and their risk of sudden death (death within three hours of beginning of symptoms) was almost six times greater.

Dr. Stamler was shocked at the results, and warned, "These findings deserve to be stressed not only because elevations of diastolic pressure in the range of 90 to 99 mm

Hg. are common in our adult population, but also because many physicians dismiss such pressures as clinically insignificant. Clearly, risk of death is far too substantial to permit complacency or injudicious neglect."

Later, the statistics from the Chicago study and the Framingham study were combined with four other similar studies done in other cities. The same deathly finger pointed to high blood pressure as the guilty factor in all the studies.

Dr. Oglesby Paul, also of Northwestern, who reported on the pooled data, said in his scientific paper, "It is not too much to say that the diagnosis, study, and treatment of mild hypertension in young and middle-aged adults constitutes one of our greatest health challenges today."

A study was also done of twenty-two thousand army officers. Findings showed that even men who had only temporary increases in blood pressures had higher death rates from circulatory and kidney diseases.

It is essential, indeed vital to your very life, to pay attention to your blood pressure.

### Other countries

The same statistics are shown wherever they are measured. The World Health Organization studied nearly eight thousand persons living in seven cities—Prague (Czechoslovakia), Hisayama and Saju (Japan), Malmo (Sweden), and Moscow, Riga, and Ryazan (U.S.S.R.). The findings: that persons with high blood pressure had a 25 percent higher prevalence of coronary heart disease than those with lower pressures.

### Even more dangerous in blacks

Just as blacks get high blood pressure more frequently and

at an earlier age, the complications seem to be more severe when they hit.

Dr. J. B. Johnson, a heart specialist in Washington, was a case in point. He knew about his blood pressure condition for many years but like so many doctors really did not take care of himself. He himself was deeply involved in a study of hypertension when he died. He must have realized that the throbbing ache behind his skull was no simple headache and must have suspected that he was experiencing the first beginnings of a stroke. Indeed, when the steering wheel seemed to fly beyond his control and he found himself suddenly crashing into a parked car, his suspicions must have been confirmed. Hours later, with his vision blurred and his breathing scratchy and labored, he died with a massive stroke.

Strokes are a particular problem, often occurring at an early age and often fatal on the first occurrence, even in teenagers.

Congestive heart failure, secondary to hypertension, is also much more severe in the black person as compared to the white person. Blacks however have a lower percentage of heart attacks.

The reason for the difference is not known; but, importantly, the high blood pressure in blacks, even though it may be worse, still responds just as well to treatment as it does in whites.

High blood pressure, in blacks or whites, is controllable.

### *What pressures give you the longest life?*

According to Edward Lew, medical director of the Metropolitan Life Insurance Company, the persons who live the very longest have pressures below 110 mm systolic and 70 mm diastolic.

# 6

# *Where to Go for Screening*

Not too long ago, we did a study in Washington that pointed up the desperate need for better detection of high blood pressure. We sent a nurse from our study group to record blood pressures in one thousand three hundred patients in our own city hospital. She found that four hundred patients (31 percent) had a high blood pressure reading. And 285 of them did not know they were hypertensive. Only *8 percent* were receiving treatment for their high blood pressures. The only place where high blood pressure was adequately measured and treated was on the medical and obstetrical services. This was in a hospital!

After this we sent high school students around to three other hospitals in Washington to take blood pressures. They went to the dermatology, genito-urinary, and orthopedic outpatient clinics where we felt blood pressures were not usually taken. We were right! High blood pressure was found in 43 to 51 percent of the patients. Only 8 percent— the same as our nurse had found—were under treatment for the disease.

Routine screening is not being done in hospitals. And it is

not being done by many physicians. Indeed, psychiatrists, dermatologists, ophthalmologists, and surgeons, for example, often do not even have a blood pressure cuff in active use.

Screening programs for detecting high blood pressure by taking blood pressures in supermarkets, churches, women's clubs, firehouses, etc., are important, but an even more important first step would be to guarantee that every person who goes to any medical or dental facility for any reason would have his blood pressure checked there.

We are not arguing against community screening programs—any and every method for detecting and treating undiagnosed hypertensives is important. It would seem more practical, however, to practice good medicine in our hospitals and clinics before going out into the community.

## *Can I get my blood pressure checked by my regular doctor?*

Yes, by all means. The American Medical Association and the government's task force on high blood pressure both recommend that testing be done in every doctor's office, in every clinic, and in every hospital as a routine measure. So you may have your blood pressure checked on a visit to any one of these.

Be sure to ask what your blood pressure reading is, and write it down so that you won't forget it.

Many physicians do not tell their patients when they have slightly elevated blood pressure on the theory that this will scare them and that the knowledge alone will drive the pressure even higher.

We believe that everyone has the right to know all about his body and what is going on inside it. And we believe that people *want* to know all the facts. Then they need not be afraid of the unknown. Nor do they need to worry about having high blood pressure because they know it can be fixed.

So do not be satisfied with a doctor's casual remark that you have a slightly elevated blood pressure and need not worry about it. Get the specifics on *how* high it is. And discuss with your doctor what specific things he suggests that you do to bring it down.

Perhaps it is only a little high, and you really don't need medication, but you want to *know* that for sure. Maybe you need to cut down your weight, or to stop smoking. Talk about it with your doctor so you know the complete picture.

And make sure to get your pressure checked again in six months to know that it has not gone higher.

### *Dental programs*

Many people see their dentists once or twice a year and may well not see doctors that often. So now dentists are considering taking blood pressure, too.

A national program for the country's one hundred twenty-one thousand dentists to screen their patients is urged by Dr. Charles L. Berman of Hackensack, New Jersey, after a pilot study in which 1,343 patients were screened in seventeen participating dental offices. About 5 percent of patients, living in a county well-served with medical care, were found to have elevated pressure, and 88 percent of them did see their doctors about it. The test was conducted by the Bergen County, New Jersey, Dental Society and Bergen County Health Department, with support from the county medical society.

If it is adopted nationally, you may well find your dentist or dental aide taking your blood pressure on your routine visits for dental care.

Says Dr. Berman, "Screening for hypertension can easily be performed at the time of a dental examination. In order to detect hypertension in its early stages, it is necessary to check a patient's blood pressure on a regular basis. The dentist is uniquely suited to do this."

Hypertension is analogous to dental caries, he says. "Both diseases cause irreparable deterioration, and both can be controlled if detected early. The difference is that undetected hypertension can cause death."

### *Where are mass free screenings available now?*

You may find a screening center in a supermarket, a bank, a special van, a school, a church, or in a clinic or hospital.

Some of the checking will be done by private groups, such as companies screening their employees, some by public agencies such as city health departments, some by voluntary organizations such as the American Heart Association.

Sometimes the screening is done in massive weekend or week-long drives, or teams will go from house to house to check the pressures of the people who live there. At other times, permanent facilities are set up. Some school systems are beginning to test all high school seniors for high blood pressure.

The government itself is not conducting screenings, but is encouraging it in every way possible. So serious is the epidemic of high blood pressure considered to be, in fact, that the National Heart and Lung Institute is conducting a special National High Blood Pressure Education Program to alert Americans about the dangers, and to encourage them to find out what their blood pressures really are. The American Medical Association, the American Heart Association, and other organizations are sponsoring similar campaigns. The main purpose is to identify the millions of people who have high pressure and don't know it, and to put them under life-saving treatment.

### *How can I find out where to go in my neighborhood?*

Watch your local newspaper and television station for announcements of special screening programs. Call your local medical society, nearest hospital, or your city health department, and ask them where free facilities are available. Or call the local office of the American Heart Association. They are carrying out a vigorous educational campaign that includes the distribution of campaign kits with educational materials to more than two hundred Heart Associations in the fifty states.

### *The Veterans Administration*

The Veterans Administration is also engaged in the search for unsuspecting victims of hypertension. In one screening of seventy thousand men in sixteen hospitals across the country, one-third were found to have high blood pressure. In this screening, pressure was considered high with a diastolic (resting) pressure of 100 to 105.

The goal of the V.A. is to expand their testing to all 168 veterans hospitals, and so eventually screen all thirty million veterans in the United States. So if you are a veteran, you may have your blood pressure taken at the nearest V.A. hospital. The program may eventually be expanded to include veterans' families.

### *Government programs*

If you work for the government, you may be eligible for free screening through your work. Several government agencies are screening or planning to screen their employees. The Health Services Administration has set up a federal employee health screening program in Washington, and plans have been made to establish others.

## The CHEC program

Another large series of surveys are presently being done by CHEC (Community Hypertension Evaluation Clinic). So far, they have already screened one hundred fifty thousand persons in nearly one hundred cities. Of these people, 28 percent have been referred to their personal physicians because of high pressure.

These screening projects are sponsored in each city by the local chapter of the American Heart Association, a local medical society, and the Ciba Pharmaceutical Company, with hundreds of volunteer workers assisting in the effort.

In New Orleans some thirty thousand people were tested in one busy weekend that was promoted and publicized with radio announcements, newspaper stories, banners flying, and Al Hirt playing his jazz trumpet. Posters were placed in shopping centers, banks, department stores, drugstores, and buses. Churches and synagogues urged their congregations to cooperate.

At forty-three schools, two thousand volunteers distributed literature, kept the lines moving, made referrals to health-care resources, and tabulated the results. Members of the National Guard ran duty tours at each school, and set up a network of communications between schools.

Of the thirty thousand people who stormed into the schools beginning at eight in the morning, an average of 28 percent had high readings and were referred to their doctors.

In San Diego, in a similar program, the teams screened fifty thousand persons, from age five up, with almost 30 percent referred to physicians. In Columbia, Maryland, 24 percent were referred. In Livingston, New Jersey, it was a whopping 40 percent.

### Aren't these percentages higher than earlier estimates?

Yes. It may well prove to be, the experts, including insurance companies, are now saying, that not one out of five, but *one out of three adults may have high blood pressure!* That means that some forty to forty-three million instead of the estimated twenty-three million Americans might have the disease.

### Neighborhood health centers

Many screening programs are being set up as a permanent part of neighborhood health centers. One such effort is Project Hi Blood, sponsored by the Wayne Miner Neighborhood Health Center in Kansas City, which operates with federal support, concentrating on the inner city, with a poor and predominantly black population. One exciting aspect that is paying off is the use of people from the area itself as community health aides to reach residents and to communicate information about high blood pressure and health problems.

In Boston, an evening walk-in service has been started by the Belmont-Watertown Community Health Association for people with hypertension who cannot take time off from work. The services are operated by an experienced public health nurse who takes blood pressures, checks weight, instructs on proper dieting and reports findings back to a physician. Whenever blood pressure is beyond normal limits, the patient is referred back to his own physician or, in the absence of a physician, is encouraged to select one, or to visit a clinic.

## The National Heart and Lung Institute testing program

The government's role in high blood pressure is basically education—to make both the public and physicians more aware of the dangers of high blood pressure and of the fact that it can be treated. But the government is sponsoring one screening and treatment program. It has been set up by the National Heart and Lung Institute in fourteen communities where about fifty thousand people have been screened so far. Of those screened, some ten thousand who have high blood pressure are entering a treatment program and will be followed for five years. One-half will be treated by their regular doctor or clinic. The other half will be treated at the program's own clinic, using the government's recommended treatment program. Both groups will be checked periodically to see whether the government's specific recommended treatment program is better than the mixed treatments given in the medical community.

## The MR. FIT program

A similar study is the Multiple Risk Factor Intervention Trial (MRFIT). MR. FIT is to determine how well coronary heart disease can be prevented by reducing the risk factors of elevated blood pressure, elevated serum cholesterol, and cigarette smoking among men aged thirty-four to fifty-four—the age of highest risk of developing coronary heart disease.

Fifteen clinical centers are in the MR. FIT program along with a central coordinating center. And currently thousands of people are coming to the centers to get help in changing their diet, giving up smoking, and taking medication to control their high blood pressure.

## Other countries

The hypertension epidemic is a world-wide one and a major concern of the World Health Organization, which has held recent meetings on the problem in Monaco, Geneva, and Göteborg.

The first step will be to determine statistics on a world-wide basis: how many people have high blood pressure, how many people know they have it, how many are receiving adequate treatment?

In some places the general population will be screened. In others, special groups will be studied: certain occupational groups, groups with different levels of income, rural versus urban.

A survey will also be done of the incidence of complications: how many people have stroke, heart disease, kidney failure.

Some of the countries involved so far include Barbados, Finland, France, Israel, Italy, Japan, Mongolia, Nigeria, Turkey, the U.S.S.R., Belgium, Sweden, and the United Kingdom.

## Who should be screened?

According to the Inter-Society Commission for Heart Disease Resources, "The population between fifteen and sixty-five years of age should be routinely screened."

We think pediatricians should routinely take blood pressure in younger children, too.

## When should you have your blood pressure taken?

Now. At the first opportunity you get. Don't wait until you

feel bad. Then, it may be too late and the damage already done.

### What if I have already had my blood pressure taken?

It depends on how long ago. Just because you had your blood pressure taken a year ago and it was normal doesn't necessarily mean it is normal now. You should get it rechecked every year.

### How complicated is the screening test?

Not complicated at all. It takes about a minute and consists of a nurse or medical assistant wrapping a cuff around your arm, pumping air into it, then letting the air out and listening to your pulse with a stethoscope. No pain, no needle—just a brisk pressure on your upper arm.

The system is so simple that in Italy there are popular street machines where you can measure your blood pressure for a fee.

The apparatus used to measure blood pressure is called a sphygmomanometer (sfig'-mo-mah-no'-me-tor).

### Sphygmo who?

Sphygmomanometer. It's a device consisting of a cloth bag or cuff that is wrapped around your arm above the elbow, and a rubber bulb to inflate the bag with air. All of this is attached to a column of mercury similar to a thermometer that gets pushed up by the pressure of the air in the bag.

The rubber bulb is squeezed until air pressure stops the blood flow through the main artery in your arm. As the air pressure is eased, a stethoscope picks up the sound of pulsing blood, a distinct thudding noise. The level of mercury when you hear this first sound is the systolic or beating pressure. As more air is released, the thudding sound fades out. The level of the mercury column when the thudding sound disappears is the diastolic or resting pressure. Both readings are expessed in millimeters of mercury, usually written by its chemical symbol as mm Hg.

## *Is it difficult to measure blood pressure?*

No. Most people can be trained quite quickly to take fairly accurate readings. A doctor is certainly not needed. In fact, we have taught our kids to take our blood pressures at home.

In the screening programs, doctors seldom take the blood pressures. The job is done by nurses, medical assistants, or other properly trained aides. In many areas, high school students are doing an excellent job.

## *What should I do if a check shows my reading is high?*

First, have it rechecked, by your doctor or at a clinic. There could be temporary reasons why one reading was elevated. You may be one of the people whose blood pressure goes up just from being tested. You may have been under some other temporary strain. Or, you may truly have high blood pressure. For your health's sake, you want to be sure, either way.

No doctor will treat a patient for a single elevated reading, but one should give some importance to it. The data from the study done in Framingham, Massachusetts, showed that one elevated reading above 160 mm Hg. systolic pressure was associated with a 50 percent increase in the incidence of stroke.

If you should have a single elevated reading, don't be

alarmed. But you should keep frequent track of your pressure in the future for other high readings.

### How many readings
### are recommended for confirmation?

Most physicians prefer three readings, on different days, for an indication that your pressure is *persistently* high.

### And if it is?

Then you should have a good physical examination and tests to try to find out what is causing your elevated pressure, and to put you under the most effective treatment.

### Okay, but what is "high" pressure?

Task Force One in the government's national education program suggests that anyone with a reading of 160/95 or higher be referred to a clinic or his physician, for a decision as to whether treatment is needed. The World Health Organization and the American Medical Association also use 160/95 for referral.

This referral does not necessarily mean you have high blood pressure. You can't tell from one reading. It simply means you should have it checked further.

### If my pressure is high,
### how soon should I see a doctor?

An appointment for further evaluation and possible treatment should be made within twenty-four to forty-eight hours. High blood pressure is an important health situation.

If you put off the appointment, you might not get around to doing it. If your screening test indicates you may have high blood pressure, make an appointment right then in the center for a further check, or pick up the phone as soon as you get home and make an appointment with your own doctor.

### The need for follow-up

It doesn't do any good to find out that you have high blood pressure if you don't do anything about it. One of the biggest problems faced by the screening programs is getting people to follow through, to go to their doctor or clinic for further evaluation when their pressure is high.

Sometimes more than half of the people referred to a doctor fail to show up for further check or treatment. One thing that seems to help is an immediate appointment. In our clinics in Washington, for example, when we suggested that people have a further checkup in a week, only 50 percent did so. Now we say, "Can you come back this afternoon or tomorrow?" and 95 percent of them show up.

"Getting the patient to the physician and persuading him to continue treatment are the two biggest problems we have," says Dr. Joseph A. Wilber, who is involved in a large screening program in Atlanta. "If an elevated blood pressure level just made one feel sick, most of the problems in community control would be solved."

But high blood pressure doesn't give you signs until damage has been done, so see to it that you do go in for further evaluation if your test reading is high.

### A second screening

Some programs are using a second screening before people with a high pressure are referred to a physician.

Those people referred for a second screen receive three measurements of blood pressure. Those who have pressures of less than 140/90 are considered as needing no further evaluation at the time. Those with pressures greater than 140/90 are given further evaluation.

### At what reading are most people given treatment?

A rule of thumb is a diastolic pressure of 105. Although many doctors would start treatment at a pressure a good deal lower.

The Task Force of the government's High Blood Pressure Education Committee recommends the following:

The person with a diastolic pressure of 105 or above should be treated. (However, he should have his pressure taken two or three times to make sure this is a true reading and he is not being falsely diagnosed.)

Anyone having a reading above 120 diastolic on the initial screening should begin medication *immediately*, even before further tests are done. Such a person is considered in imminent danger of a stroke or other complication so that immediate treatment—that day—is needed.

### What about the person who is only mildly hypertensive, that is, has a diastolic pressure of 90 to 104?

First, he should have a second reading taken, then meet with his doctor.

Some doctors believe that a person with mild high blood pressure should be treated; others prefer to wait and carefully watch the blood pressure to see what it does.

Usually the doctor takes into account other risk factors. For instance, he is more likely to prescribe medicines for you if you are young, black, overweight, smoke, or have a family history of high blood pressure, strokes, or heart disease.

We will go into more detail on how it is determined whether treatment is needed in the next two chapters.

## *Planning a screening program*

If you are involved in planning a screening program for your place of business or for your town, there are a number of things you must take into account.

First, the local medical society must be brought into the planning stage. A screening program is only as good as its follow-up, only as good as the treatment that results from it, so you must have the cooperation of the physicians in the community.

In fact, at the planning sessions, you should have representatives of the medical society, heart association, public health department, local hospitals, nursing organizations, city officials and, most important, neighborhood community leaders. Local representatives of pharmaceutical companies will often provide training aids and educational materials for distribution in the program.

Newspaper editors and radio and television editors need to be briefed to publicize the event.

Nurses, medical assistants, and other volunteers must be checked to be sure that they are taking blood pressures correctly, and a refresher training course should be set up. Volunteers need to be instructed in detail on how to advise people about their readings and to make immediate appointments for further evaluation if readings are high.

As you plan your program, remember you don't need to build a building for screening purposes. Use existing facilities. Temporary testing centers can be set up almost anywhere, from schools to shopping centers. Permanent testing facilities can find a home in a corner of a clinic, hospital, or medical centers.

The American Heart Association has a community organization guide to help you start a high blood pressure program.

# 7

# *Going to the Doctor*

Let's say you've been for a checkup as part of an examination for an insurance policy and have been told you have high blood pressure—more people find out that way than any other. Or you may have been told at a neighborhood screening center or at work.

In either event, you've been advised to see a doctor for further evaluation. What should you expect?

### *The purpose of the visit*

This visit is to evaluate the exact status of your blood pressure.

The doctor will determine if you really do have high blood pressure, and if so, how severe it is. He will determine whether there has been any damage done by high pressure to your brain, heart, eyes, or kidneys. He will determine whether you need treatment, and if so, what kind.

He will want to identify any other health problems you may have that could affect the high blood pressure or the treatment approach in any way.

He will want to identify any other risk factors for stroke or heart attack that might be present, such as overweight, or whether or not you are a smoker.

## Confirming your number

As mentioned earlier most physicians believe that at least three blood pressure readings should be taken on different occasions before they can say for sure that a person has high blood pressure.

Many things can affect your blood pressure—the time of day, being cold, running for a bus, being nervous or afraid, physical discomfort, pain, body position, a sudden loud noise, strange surroundings, your reaction to the person taking the measurement, or a full bladder. Before your doctor starts you on medicines that you will probably be taking for the rest of your life, he wants to make sure that you really *need* them, that you don't just have a falsely high reading.

## How your blood pressure is taken

After being checked in by the receptionist, you will be shown to a small room and asked to be seated or to lie down. After you have relaxed for about five minutes, the pressure is taken on both arms and recorded and compared. Another reading is usually taken after you have been standing for a minute or so.

Accuracy in these readings is so important that special training programs are set up to train people to take blood pressures correctly. And special steps are taken, such as having wider cuffs for fat people and narrow cuffs for children, to ensure accurate readings.

### *The one most important thing for you to do*

The single most important thing that you can do in seeing the doctor is—relax. High blood pressure or not, worrying isn't going to help. If you find out you *don't* have high pressure, that will be good news. If you *do* have it, there's still no need to worry because high blood pressure is a disease you can do something about. It can be controlled.

But there's an even more practical reason to relax. And that is, if you are anxious and tense about being in the doctor's office or about having your pressure taken, it can drive your blood pressure reading way up, making the doctor think that you have high blood pressure when you really don't.

This false high reading is such a problem that some doctors say as many as 30 to 40 percent of their patients end up with falsely high readings on their first visit. So to find the true number, we take several measurements, one or two at the beginning of a visit, another at the end when the patient is more relaxed. Some doctors have a patient come back several times a week for repeated recordings, hoping the patient will relax.

With some patients we feel as if we might as well throw the blood pressure cuff out the window. These are the types whose usually normal diastolic blood pressure of 85 will zoom up to 130 the moment they walk into the examining room. One doctor has threatened to start serving cocktails in his waiting room to help people relax when they come in. Another tells anxious patients to breathe deeply for several minutes.

Dr. Maurice Sokolow, chief of the cardiovascular division of the University of California in San Francisco, often uses a portable blood pressure apparatus for home recordings to find a person's true pressure. Several of his patients who had been diagnosed in the office for years as having high blood pressure turned out to be perfectly normal.

So it is important for you to relax when you go to have a checkup. Take your time, leave home early so you don't have to rush, read a book or something while you wait, and try to keep calm, cool and unruffled.

### Talk to your doctor

Another important point in feeling at ease is to feel free to discuss with your doctor anything that might be bothering you. If you have a question, ask it; don't stew about it—and perhaps raise your blood pressure.

Dr. Edward Freis, coordinator of a famous study conducted by the Veterans Administration that proved drugs do work in controlling high pressure, says one major problem is that after taking a reading "some physicians will say nothing about the results of the reading and ask the patient to return in a week for additional examination. The mysterious silence in regard to the blood pressure level and the ominous request to return practically assure a brisk pressure response on the next visit."

Talk about your problems. Ask questions. Get your actual number. And relax.

### The basic tests

The tests and measurements that are done on a first visit for possible hypertension are simple ones. Blood pressure, height, and weight.

If your pressure reading is normal, you probably will have no other tests, but will be asked to come back in a year for another check on your pressure.

If your pressure is above normal, then you will have a small sample of blood taken from your arm for some lab work, and you will be asked for a urine specimen for other tests.

Either at this visit or a second, your doctor will do a complete medical history and physical examination. And an x-ray and electrocardiogram will be taken to check on the size and function of your heart.

## The medical history

When the nurse or doctor takes your medical history, asking you questions about your family's medical background and your own medical problems, past and present, it is important to answer all the questions completely and accurately. This is no time to fudge on birth dates, give in to false modesty, or pretend that you are a superman with a perfect medical history. Tell your doctor *everything*, even if it seems embarrassing. No matter how embarrassing it may be to you, he's heard it a hundred times before. We're looking for the facts, and all of them.

It may seem like a drag to go through the long history, and when he asks you about your past illnesses or present problems, you may think it's a waste of time. Well, it isn't, because these facts are all important in assessing your present condition; in addition, they are necessary in choosing the right drug for you.

## Taking your own medical history

To save you and your doctor time, and to give you an opportunity to think through your answers so they are completely accurate, we have reproduced here a list of questions adapted from a medical history form used by the Hypertension Detection and Follow-up Program sponsored by the National Heart and Lung Institute.

Read the questions and make a list of the symptoms that apply to you. Keep this as part of your permanent medical record, and take it with you to your doctor for your next checkup.

Has any close relative (father, mother, brothers, sisters, children) ever had heart disease, high blood pressure, stroke, diabetes, or kidney disease?

Has any relative ever died from stroke or heart attack at an early age?

Do you have any conditions or health problems at the present time?

Has a doctor ever told you that you had kidney stones or other kidney trouble? Gout? Cirrhosis or liver disease? Tuberculosis? Diabetes? Intestinal bleeding or ulcers?

Have you ever had a kidney or bladder infection or an injury to the kidneys?

In the past several months, have you been troubled with skin rash or bruising? Headaches so bad that you had to stop what you were doing? Faintness or light-headedness when you stand up quickly? Ringing in the ears? Your heart beating fast or skipping beats? Blacking out or losing consciousness? Swelling or tenderness of your breasts? Recurrent stomach pains? Waking up too early and having difficulty getting back to sleep? Stools black or tarry? Blood in your stools? Decreased sexual ability? Feeling so depressed or sad that it interfered with your work, recreation, or sleep?

Do you usually have to go to the bathroom in the middle of the night?

Are you overweight?

Have you ever been pregnant? How many miscarriages or stillbirths? Have seizures or convulsions occurred during any pregnancy? Has high blood pressure or toxemia complicated any pregnancy?

Are you currently taking birth control pills?

Have you ever had any pain or discomfort in your chest? Ever had any pressure or heaviness in your chest?

Do you get pain (or discomfort) when you walk uphill or

hurry? When you walk at an ordinary pace on the level?

Do you get pain in either leg on walking? When you are standing still or sitting?

Do you ever get shortness of breath that requires you to stop and rest? Do you get it walking on level ground or climbing a single flight of stairs? When you are lying down flat? Does it improve when you sit up, or do you use extra pillows at night to prevent it?

Do you usually cough first thing in the morning on getting up or on first going outdoors in the winter? Do you frequently cough or bring up phlegm during the day—or at night—in the winter?

Does your chest ever sound wheezing or whistling? Have you ever had attacks of shortness of breath with wheezing?

Do you smoke cigarettes? More than a pack a day?

Has any medication ever caused you to have a skin rash or other kind of allergic reaction?

Have you taken any medications or drugs or treatments, including special diet, lately?

### *The physical examination*

In addition to knowing just how high your blood pressure is, your doctor will want to know what effect, if any, it has had on the blood vessels, and on various organs. So he will pay particular attention to these as he does your physical examination.

He will carefully study your heart since it is a frequent target organ for damage from high blood pressure. He'll look for heart enlargement, listen for abnormal sounds, and study the electrocardiogram results for signs of heart disease. He'll listen to your chest and look for swelling around the ankles that would indicate poor heart function.

He will also check the state of your arteries, looking for abnormal sounds called "thrills" that can be felt or heard when there is damage. He'll check to see if you have a strong pulse that is equal on both of your arms and legs.

He will look at your eyes, which are not only your windows on the world but also windows for the doctor to see inside you. When he shines a light into your eye, telling you to "look straight ahead," and peers intently at your eye, he is looking through the opening of your pupil to blood vessels in the back of the eye. If he sees a constriction of the arteries, or arteriosclerosis, or tiny hemorrhages, it gives a clue to what might be happening elsewhere in your body.

He'll check your nerve reflexes and look for other signs that might indicate brain damage.

He'll feel your abdomen to check for enlargement or other abnormality of the kidneys.

## Laboratory examinations

The routine laboratory examinations that are recommended for people with hypertension are standard tests available in every lab and relatively inexpensive.

Your blood will be checked for potassium, sugar, urea (a test for kidney function), and cholesterol.

Your urine will be tested for sugar, albumin, and for signs of infection.

## What about more extensive testing?

Unless the doctor suspects some special complication or that you have one of the more rare forms of hypertension, there is no need for extensive and expensive testing.

And yet this is one of the greatest dilemmas of the doctor in practice today and a subject of controversy in the medical profession. To treat without knowing the cause of a problem is against medical training. Students in medical school are taught to reach a definite diagnosis before starting treatment. But with high blood pressure, the general rule with most doctors is to treat first, and only do further tests if the patient doesn't respond.

The important thing is to get the high blood pressure under control, not to do a lot of fancy tests.

As one doctor says, "If my daughter were coming to me, and she was over forty years old, truly all I would do would be the urine tests, blood tests, x-ray and EKG."

### How can you tell if you have the kind of hypertension that can be permanently cured by surgery—the 10 percent?

If you have this kind, instead of the "essential hypertension" that occurs most often, it will gradually, despite medicine, get worse. Or there will be other signs that turn up during the physical examination suggesting one of the rare forms. Once your doctor suspects that you have one of these kinds of hypertension, he will do the more extensive tests to establish a definite diagnosis and the proper treatment procedure.

### What are the recommendations of the government's task force on testing?

The experts on the government's advisory committee say that the pre-treatment examination, whether done by a doctor or his assistant, should include:

Height and weight.
Examination of the eyes.
Listening to the lungs for signs of heart failure.
Examination of the heart for increased size, murmurs and arrhythmias.

Examination of the extremities for edema and neurologic deficits.

Laboratory and other tests, they say, should include:

Electrocardiogram.
Chest x-ray.
Urinalysis for protein, hemoglobin, and glucose (Dipstick).
Blood urea nitrogen or creatinine.
Blood sugar.
Serum potassium.
Serum cholesterol.
Uric acid.

## What happens next?

Your doctor will look over all the findings: the facts gathered from the history and the physical, the laboratory results, plus additional things you may have told him, and will decide what looks like the best course for you to follow.

*If your blood pressure is below 90 diastolic and 140 systolic,* he will happily tell you your blood pressure is fine, and that you should return for a regular checkup, including blood pressure reading, every year, just as everyone should.

*If your diastolic pressure is above 90, but below 105,* the doctor will decide whether you should have treatment based on all the other factors he has discovered. The younger you are, for example, the more likely he is to start treatment, since high blood pressure is especially dangerous when it begins before age 40. The higher the blood pressure and the younger the patient, the higher the priority for treatment.

He is also more likely to treat you if you have target organ damage of the eyes, heart, brain, or kidneys; if you are a man, since high blood pressure seems to affect men more severely than women; if you have a family history of high blood pressure, stroke, or heart disease; if you have a high blood level of cholesterol; or if you have diabetes.

All of these conditions tend to add some risk to the high blood pressure picture, and so make treatment more necessary at this intermediate blood pressure level than would ordinarily be necessary.

If none of these factors applies to you, then you probably do not need treatment, and should simply be sure to have a yearly checkup and yearly blood pressure reading.

### What if your blood pressure is over 105?

Then, according to the National Hypertension Information and Education Advisory Committee, your doctor definitely should recommend treatment.

The ideal goal of treatment, they say, should be "to bring the diastolic blood pressure below 90 mm Hg.," with a diastolic of less than 100 mm Hg., however, being considered acceptable.

### How urgent is treatment?

In general, the higher the blood pressure, the more urgent is the need to start treatment immediately. But remember there are all those other factors that may make treatment more urgent or less urgent than a mere number.

The urgency of treatment depends on the state of your blood vessels; the amount of damage done to your heart, brain, or kidneys. And it depends on the other risk factors that hazard a heart attack or stroke, such as whether you are fat, whether you smoke, whether you have high cholesterol or diabetes.

As Dr. John H. Laragh of Columbia University in New York says, "You don't live or die because of a number. You've got to plug the number into the situation."

If you are twenty years old with a diastolic reading of 95 to 100, that is alarming. But it is not so alarming in a person aged sixty.

You are sick or well according to the amount of blood vessel damage you have. Your heart is a pump, your arteries are pipes to distribute blood. If, despite a high reading, your pipes are normal, and your pump is normal, we just have to say that your blood pressure is high right now, and make an appointment for a recheck in a few days. If high pressure is a regular thing, if the heart is weakened and enlarged, if your kidneys are bad, that is what kills you.

But you should know your number, so you know what your own individual situation is from year to year.

### *The task force score sheet*

How can a doctor determine risk for a particular patient, how can he tell just how urgent it is for a patient to have medical treatment to control pressure? One of the government's task forces on high blood pressure was concerned with just this problem.

The task force came up with this score sheet. It was actually designed for physicians to use in evaluating their patients, but you, too, can use it to evaluate your own situation.

What is your diastolic blood pressure?
105 to 120 = 3 points
120 to 140 = 6 points
over 140   = 9 points
What is your racial background?
Being black = 1 point
Are you more or less than 40 years old?
Being less than age 40 = 1 point
Are you male or female?
Being male = 1 point

Have you ever had heart failure?
Heart failure = 1 point

Add up your total number of points.

It is the view of the task force that the higher the point total, the greater the urgency of therapy, and treatment should be considered urgent for subjects with six or more points.

## The next step

Choosing the right medicine for you is something you and your doctor have to work out together. He will choose the medicine, but it will be up to you to report back to him on how it makes you feel so that he can be sure to prescribe the medication that suits you best.

The drug to start with is pretty standard—a thiazide diuretic. It usually does the job of getting pressure down to normal in about 80 or 90 percent of patients. But if not, then your doctor will try other drugs. We will outline the medication procedure, and how you can work with your doctor in trying them, in the next chapter.

## Later visits

High blood pressure is not a disease that you simply treat once and cure. It requires lifelong treatment. So you will be going back to the doctor on a regular basis for checkups.

These checkups are important for several reasons:

First, your doctor needs to make sure that your blood pressure is properly under control. Remember, you can't tell how high your pressure is by the way you feel.

Second, he may want to adjust your medicine. Your blood pressure may have gotten worse, or it may have improved. Or you may be having side effects that can be eliminated with a different drug.

Third, he wants to keep a close watch on your heart, brain, and kidneys to make sure no damage is developing that you're not aware of. Remember, it's not the blood pressure itself that you're concerned about, it's the damage it can do to other organs. To *prevent* that damage is what treatment is all about.

When you leave your doctor's office, make sure you know when he wants you back. It's a good idea to make an appointment right then.

And be sure to keep it.

### Should the doctor tell me my blood pressure number?

Three doctors were discussing this question while making a tape recording on hypertension. One doctor, Theodore Cooper, who heads the government's National Heart and Lung Institute in Washington, and also heads the inter-agency task force investigations, said, "Many physicians have some hesitancy in telling the patient his blood pressure number. I repeatedly have recommended that the patient ask the doctor to tell him his blood pressure, and to write it down."

Dr. Mitchell Perry, professor of medicine at Washington University School of Medicine in St. Louis, said, "Now, when we can lower virtually everybody's blood pressure, a patient has a right to know what his pressure is, and he has a right to know what his continuing pressure is—in other words, how effective therapy is. As a matter of fact, in most of my own patients, I carry this to the next step and give him a sphygmomanometer and have him take his own blood pressure at home."

Dr. Richard Hurley, vice president for medical affairs of the American Heart Association, agreed. "What you're really talking about," he said, "is involving the patient in his own care. If he knows what his pressure is, if he knows what happens, he can respond. He knows what's going on. He is motivated to keep up treatment. We've not used the patients as much as we should in their own health care."

We agree completely with these three leading doctors.

### What if you don't think you have high blood pressure, but are just going to the doctor for some other reason?

Any time you go to any doctor or any clinic or any hospital for a first visit, *your blood pressure should be taken.* That includes not only a visit to a doctor for a complete physical examination, but it also includes first visits to an obstetrician, a dermatologist, a psychiatrist, or a doctor who removes a wart from your left little toe.

This policy has been formally stated by the American Medical Association, and has also been backed by the National Medical Association, the American Heart Association, the Citizen's Committee Against High Blood Pressure, and the government's task force making recommendations. Obviously, if you are going to a psychiatrist every week for therapy or are getting that left toe wart treated every other week, you don't need to have your blood pressure taken each time. But on a first visit, or if the doctor hasn't seen you for a year, no matter what his specialty, he (or his assistant) should take your blood pressure. If he doesn't do it, feel free to request it.

### How often should I see my doctor?

If you are in the group of people who have blood pressure of 105 to 120 diastolic, then you will usually be seeing your physician every two weeks or so at the beginning of treatment. By the time it is under control, if you have no symptoms or problems that need discussing, you can see him every two to four months.

If your blood pressure is higher than 120, the average interval between visits at first is one week. If your blood pressure is normal, you should see your doctor once a year for a blood pressure reading.

# 8

# *The Newest Drugs to Treat High Blood Pressure*

In 1964 a history-making study was begun in the United States that completely changed the outlook of people with high blood pressure.

The study was done by a team of doctors in seventeen Veterans Administration hospitals across the country. There were thirty doctors and three statisticians working on the project, headed by Dr. Edward D. Freis, of the V.A. hospital in Washington, D.C. They took hundreds of men with moderately severe high blood pressure, and divided them into two groups, carefully selected to be evenly matched by age, race, and other characteristics. Then one group of men was treated with drugs for high blood pressure and the other group was not.

The results were dramatic. Of the men *not* receiving high blood pressure medicine, there were four deaths in the test period and twenty-seven serious heart attacks or strokes. And there was some eye damage, congestive heart failure and kidney damage. Of the men taking the medicine, there were *no* deaths and only *one* stroke. It was so obvious that the pills did prevent heart failure and strokes and did save lives that, even though the study was not finished, the doctors felt they had to immediately give the untreated group the medicines too.

Later the same kind of study was done of the veterans who had less severe high blood pressure. There were the same kinds of striking results.

Before these studies were done, most doctors questioned whether high blood pressure medicines really did any good on a long term basis. Now it was unquestionably proved that pills could significantly and effectively prevent the crippling complications of high blood pressure. It was an important finding, and for it Dr. Freis was given one of the highest honors in medicine—the Lasker Award.

As Dr. Mitchell Perry, part of the Veterans Administration team, comments: "Before, when a patient's blood pressure was up, we didn't really know whether treating it would do any good. Now, for the first time, we can say that treatment will do some good."

### What drugs were used in the V.A. study?

Three of them, sometimes alone, sometimes in combination. They were a thiazide diuretic, reserpine, and hydralazine. Now we have even more drugs.

### Have there been other studies to show the value of treatment with drugs?

Yes, several. Probably the most impressive statistics are those from insurance companies where data gathered for years from several million people show that the person with high blood pressure who takes pills lives years longer than the person with high blood pressure who does not take pills. The difference is so striking that many insurance companies will reduce their premiums if you take pills to keep your blood pressure under control. If your blood pressure has been controlled, e.g., distolic pressure under 90 mm Hg. for four years, you are as insurable (no extra permiums) as though you never had high blood pressure. Now that should prove to you in dollars and cents how important controlling blood pressure is! In fact, the lowered rates can save you hundreds, even thousands, of dollars over the years.

### *How much can drugs lower your blood pressure?*

The ideal goal we work for is to get your diastolic pressure down to under 90 mm Hg. without side effects. In most cases, we can do it. If a particular drug causes unpleasant side effects, we will change it. With patience on both our parts, we will get your blood pressure under 90 and have you feeling fine.

### *What pills are used now?*

There are several kinds, and they act three different ways.

The one most often used is thiazide. It acts as a diuretic, that is, it flushes the excess fluid from your body by causing you to excrete more salt and more water in your urine. It is the thiazides that first revolutionized the treatment of high blood pressure and made it possible for the person with high blood pressure to have moderate amounts of salt.

Then there are drugs that act directly on the tiny arterioles which constrict to produce high blood pressure, causing them to relax.

Another group of drugs acts on the nervous system. They block the nerves that go to the blood vessels.

More medicines are being developed and tested by pharmaceutical companies.

## *Drugs for high blood pressure*

Here is a summary of the types of high blood pressure drugs in use today.

### ORAL DIURETICS

The diuretics can be classified into three general groups: (1) the thiazides and related diuretics; (2) the so-called loop diuretics; and (3) the potassium-sparing diuretics.

1. *Thiazides and related diuretics*: The thiazides and related compounds (chlorthalidone or quinethazone) are the cornerstones of high blood pressure treatment. They are used as sole therapy in patients with mild hypertension and, in patients whose hypertension is not controlled by diuretics alone, they are used with other drugs. About the only patients they don't work for are those who have kidney disease or kidney failure. The thiazides work very well, and their side effects are mild. There are no real contraindications to using a thiazide diuretic, with the possible exception of those who are allergic to them or have severe gout. With most thiazides you must take two pills a day, but one, called chlorthalidone, is longer acting and can be taken just once a day.

2. *Loop diuretics*: A "loop diuretic" is one that acts on the parts of the kidneys, the loops of Henle, that are so important in the filtering of body fluids and production of urine. The loop diuretics are about twenty times more potent than the thiazides and cause even more excretion of water and salt than the thiazides do. They are usually used in treatment of patients who have kidney damage or when thiazides have failed to lower a patient's pressure. Side effects, like those of thiazides, are infrequent and usually mild.

3. *Potassium-sparing diuretics*: There is a special group of diuretics that eliminate sodium and water and produce a drop in blood pressure similar to the thiazides but do not

lower potassium as the thiazides do. These drugs are usually added to the thiazides when the thiazides have caused excessive loss of potassium. They are not potent enough to be substituted for the thiazides.

RESERPINE

Reserpine is one of the Rauwolfia compounds, first discovered in tree roots. It is absolutely contraindicated in patients who have a history of depression or psychosis, peptic ulcer, or chronic sinusitis, since it can make these conditions worse, and it probably should not be given to patients who are obese because it increases the appetite, making it more difficult for the patient to reduce.

METHYLDOPA

This drug is most useful in patients whose blood pressure is not satisfactorily controlled with a thiazide and reserpine combination. It is especially good in patients who have kidney failure or who have uremia. It should not be used in patients who have liver disease.

HYDRALAZINE

Hydralazine is a drug that lowers blood pressure by relaxing the smooth muscles of the tiny arterioles so that they no longer contract to drive up the pressure. Hydralazine is frequently used as a third drug to be added to the treatment of patients who do not respond to a combination of thiazide and reserpine, or thiazide and methyldopa. Hydralazine, when given by itself, tends to cause a fast heartbeat and so should be used with caution in patients who have the chest pains of angina. The slowing heart action of reserpine makes the reserpine-hydralazine combination a good one.

GUANETHIDINE

This is a very powerful drug. It inhibits the production of one of the powerful pressure-raising hormones of the adrenal gland. Guanethidine stops the production of this compound and so may lower blood pressure drastically. In so doing, it sometimes causes too *low* a blood pressure and therefore must be given with great caution particularly at the beginning. In addition to the low blood pressure, guanethidine can also produce diarrhea and failure of ejaculation. The drug is therefore used only for severe, serious hypertension rather than mild or moderate pressure.

## Drugs in other countries

There are a number of other drugs that have been approved for use in Europe, but so far are not available in the United States.

In Great Britain, for example, patients are being helped by a drug called practolol. It lowers blood pressure and also relieves the chest pain of angina pectoris by blocking the actions of adrenalin.

Another drug in use in Great Britain since 1964 is guanoxan, a powerful reducer of blood pressure. It was available in this country for a while, but then the Food and Drug Administration banned it because it caused liver problems in some people who took it. British doctors are aware of the liver problems, but they take the view that for the people who do not respond to other high blood pressure medicine, the risk of liver problems is small compared to the risk of heart disease and stroke if the blood pressure is not lowered.

The only way to legally use either practolol or guanoxan is to live in Europe.

## A new drug

Diazoxide is the name of a new drug that has been released for treating dangerously high blood pressure and high blood pressure emergencies. It's a fast-acting anti-hypertensive medicine that is used so far only in hospitals where the patient can be carefully watched. It's not for routine, day-to-day treatment of high blood pressure, but for treating such conditions as malignant hypertension or for emergencies when the blood pressure has sky-rocketed to dangerous heights. Then it's injected rapidly into a vein in one large dose.

In clinical tests on one thousand patients, 95 percent were helped by the drug in an emergency situation.

There are other drugs available for treating high blood pressure emergencies but none are as effective and simple to give as diazoxide.

The drug should be given in combination with a diuretic to ensure adequate urinary output.

In certain instances, the drug is given to patients who are not responding well to other drugs. Continuously controlling the arterial pressure with diazoxide and ensuring a good output of urine with a diuretic over a two- to three-week period has frequently re-established the patient's response to simple drugs which has been lost previously.

Mrs. E.W. is a case in point. We were unable to control her blood pressure with full doses of guanethidine, hydralazine, and a diuretic. She was losing her vision and her kidney function was deteriorating. We hospitalized her and continuously controlled her blood pressure with diazoxide, using as the indication for further diazoxide a rise of diastolic blood pressure above 100 mm Hg. A good output of urine was maintained with furosemide, one of the more potent diuretics. After a single injection of the diazoxide kept her blood pressure down for twenty-four hours, we discontinued this intensive therapy and placed her back on the pills she was taking before. Much to our delight she responded beautifully. As a matter of fact, it was not necessary to re-start the guanethidine. Her blood pressure remained controlled on the hydralazine and diuretics.

### How does a doctor determine which patient should get which drugs?

First we determine whether you have mild hypertension, moderate, or severe disease, and whether you have any damage yet to your heart, blood vessels, kidneys, or brain. And we evaluate other risk factors, such as obesity, family history, smoking habits, and level of cholesterol.

In mild and moderate hypertension, 80 percent of the people only need to take a pill or two a day to be perfectly all right.

If high blood pressure is more severe, or has been present a long time, then a person usually needs more than one kind of drug each day, and probably needs to do more than just take pills. He may, for example, need to reduce the amounts of salt and cholesterol in his diet and to stop smoking.

The milder the degree of vascular disease, the simpler the treatment. The more severe the vascular disease, the more complicated the treatment.

Also your doctor needs to test how the medicines work in your particular case. People react differently to drugs. What worked for Aunt Susie may not be best for you.

And he needs to study your medical history. If you have a background of episodes of serious depression, if you have sinus trouble, or if you're obese, he shouldn't give you reserpine.

Here is a list of various medical conditions and the drugs to be avoided if you have them.

| CONDITION | DRUGS TO BE AVOIDED OR USED WITH CAUTION |
|---|---|
| Asthma | Propranolol |
| Cerebral vascular disease | Guanethidine, hydralazine |
| Collagen diseases | Hydralazine |
| Congestive heart failure | Propranolol |

| | |
|---|---|
| Coronary artery disease | Guanethidine, hydralazine |
| Diabetes mellitus | Diuretics |
| Gout | Diuretics |
| Liver disease | Methyldopa, triamterene |
| Mental depression | Reserpine |
| Migraine | Hydralazine |
| Peptic ulcer | Reserpine |
| Renal insufficiency | Spironolactone, triamterene |
| Sinus trouble | Reserpine |

### *Should the high blood pressure patient ever be hospitalized?*

A person with a very high pressure can be in real danger. Doctors vary in determining at what point a patient should be hospitalized. They do say this: that any patient who has a diastolic pressure over 120 should have his pressure lowered immediately. This does not usually require hospitalization. But if his pressure can't be lowered on the outside, then he certainly should be hospitalized.

If a person has over 140 diastolic pressure, it is extremely dangerous and he should be hospitalized immediately.

### *What about the person with only mild hypertension?*

Expert opinions vary. Scientists still aren't sure whether long term use of drugs is necessary for people with mildly high blood pressure. The government's task force recommends definite treatment at a pressure of 105 or higher, with anything between 90 and 104 being decided by the individual physician. The person above 90 or 95, they say, needs to be carefully watched, but does not necessarily need treatment.

Some doctors like to round things off with an easy-to-remember number and say that everyone with diastolic pressure over 100 should be treated.

Actually, no definite statement can be made about the management of patients whose diastolic blood pressure averages between 90 and 104 mm Hg. on repeated visits. Usually the doctor takes into account other risk factors. For instance, he is more likely to prescribe medicines for the person who is younger than 45, or black, or overweight, or who smokes, or has heart or kidney damage, or has relatives who have died of strokes or heart disease. The more of these factors pertain to you, the more likely it is that you should have treatment even though your high blood pressure is only mild.

If there is neither a positive family history nor evidence of organic damage, little will be lost with a one-year period of observation without treatment. During this period (as with all hypertensive patients), loss of weight, lowering the serum cholesterol level and the giving up of smoking should be encouraged when applicable, and the patient should be advised to have his blood pressure checked frequently, at least every six months, to make sure that it has not gone up further.

### How does the doctor know how much medicine to give you?

Usually he uses what is called a "stepped-care" program. He begins with a small dose of the mildest drug, that is, a thiazide, to see how well that works, then increases the dose if needed. If the blood pressure still has not gone down to normal, he may add, one after another, additional drugs as needed, starting each at low dosage levels and increasing the dose if necessary to do the job. This is one reason for keeping in touch with your doctor so he can periodically check your pressure and see if he needs to step up the dosage or can reduce it. The more he can keep the drug dosage down, and the fewer pills you take, the better off you are and the fewer side effects you are likely to have. Sometimes several medicines are combined in one pill so you don't have to take so many pills.

## *The recommended stepped-care program*

For the person who has a blood pressure (diastolic) of 105 to 140, the government's task force on high blood pressure treatment recommends the following to physicians: step one, give the patient thiazide. If that doesn't work, go to step two of adding one more medicine, either reserpine, methyldopa, or hydralazine. If that doesn't work, add a third drug.

## *What if I feel worse than I did before I took the pills?*

Strangely enough, this sometimes happens. You sometimes feel bad while your body is adjusting itself to the medication or to the lowered blood pressure. Or you may be having side effects caused by pills.

## *What are the side effects?*

Some people have no ill effects. Others do. In general, the milder the anti-hypertensive medication, the fewer the side effects. You see the great advantage, therefore, of discovering blood pressure in its early stage, when treatment is usually simple and without side effects.

J.D., a forty-five-year-old executive, came into my office several months ago reporting hypertension discovered three weeks earlier. He had applied recently for an insurance policy which necessitated a physical examination. His last physical examination had been twelve years ago. He had no symptoms at all, however.

Physical examination revealed a blood pressure of 160/115 mm Hg. The arteries in the back of his eyes showed arteriosclerosis. His heart was normal in size and there was no fluid in the lungs or swelling of the ankles. He was started on a thiazide diuretic. In a month's time he returned feeling quite well as he had before, but his blood pressure had only fallen to 150/105 mm Hg. I changed the pill to one that combined both thiazide and reserpine.

When he was seen again in a month's time he was complaining bitterly of nasal congestion and a fair amount of fatigue. On close questioning he also admitted to strange dreams which he had never had before. There also had been a significant change in his sleeping habits. His blood pressure was now 120/90 mm Hg. It was obvious that his complaints had nothing to do with the fall in blood pressure but were due to the new drug, so I put him back on the original thiazide and substituted methyldopa for the reserpine.

When seen three weeks later, the nasal congestion, fatigue, and bad dreams had all disappeared.

Each drug has its own particular side effects. Possible side effects include such things as drowsiness, tiredness, nasal congestion, swelling of tissues, depression, heartburn, nightmares, insomnia, dry mouth, blurred vision, dizziness, constipation, diarrhea, loss of sexual drive or performance, nausea, vomiting, nervousness, or rash.

If you are taking pills for high blood pressure and you get any of these problems, you should call your doctor. In fact, a good rule is: If you feel good, keep taking your pills—if you feel bad, call your doctor.

Side effects usually become milder as time passes.

## *What about more serious side effects?*

Some occasionally occur. In general, serious toxic effects
from the drugs used are uncommon, are easily recognized,
and are easily remedied by substituting another anti-hypertensive agent for the offending drug. Don't be embarrassed
to tell your physician of every new development or symptom. All symptoms are important. And yours may represent
a side effect which can readily be remedied.

## *Tricks of the trade for battling side effects*

We must emphasize again that 80 percent of hypertensive
patients have mild or only moderately severe disease and 80
percent of these patients can be effectively treated with a
thiazide alone or a thiazide plus reserpine. This means
taking only a pill a day with almost no side effects.

Those with more severe disease need to take more potent
drugs and these drugs may cause some undesirable side
effects. Even these can be minimized, however, as follows:

Give the drug time. Side effects can be particularly pesky
during the first few weeks of taking a drug, then they seem
to level out, and sometimes even disappear.

Then, since different medicines work differently in different people, your doctor can try one of the other
medicines for high blood pressure and keep switching
around until he finds one for you that does not cause so
many side effects. It is important that you do not let the side
effects discourage you. Keep working with your doctor to
get the best combination of medicine and the best dosages
for you because it is important for you to continue your
medication.

Start treatment as early as possible. There are fewer side
effects with lower doses of drugs and with less powerful

drugs, and the earlier treatment begins, the smaller amounts of medicine are usually needed.

Work on other contributing factors. If you give up smoking and follow your doctor's advice on diet, you may not need as many pills and so can reduce side effects.

Try changing the time you take your pills. For example, if you have side effects in the morning, but have no trouble with them the rest of the day, perhaps you can experiment (on your doctor's advice only!) by regularly taking your pill later in the day. This is one of the great things about having a simple apparatus for taking blood pressure at home. You can take your blood pressure every hour for several days and determine when your pressure tends to be up and whether there are other times when it tends to be lower. Some people can work out a chart with their doctor so that they only have to take their medicines at certain times of the day.

### *If you have dizzy spells*

Sometimes your body has not yet become used to your lowered blood pressure, so you may have episodes of dizziness or weakness. This often occurs in the morning just after you get out of bed, or if you have been standing a long time, or if you suddenly stand up from a sitting position so that the blood rushes from your head. The dizziness is accentuated by hot weather, alcohol, and exercise. Advice: Avoid prolonged standing, or standing up suddenly. Don't exercise strenuously for prolonged periods in the first few weeks of a new drug. Sit or lie down if you feel dizziness coming on.

## *If you have an upset in the balance of potassium in your body*

If your mouth is dry, you're always thirsty, you feel weak, tired, drowsy, or restless, you have muscle pains or cramps, or gastrointestinal disturbances, it may mean your medicine is causing a change in sodium or potassium levels. Report these symptoms to your physician. He may want to give you a pill that helps retain potassium. Or, he may want you to take potassium supplements, or to eat foods that are especially rich in potassium.

(Potassium can taste pretty terrible. Try adding it to lemonade or other juice and sip it through the day.)

Foods high in potassium include all bran cereals, wheat germ, brown bread, apricots, peaches, cantaloupe, watermelon, orange juice, spinach, squash, potatoes, beans, peanuts, sunflower seeds, salmon, halibut, beef, ham, and molasses.

But eating foods rich in potassium really doesn't do much good and is not very practical. For instance, you would have to eat sixteen bananas or drink fourteen glasses of orange juice a day to treat a low potassium level.

Cutting down your intake of salt will help protect you from loss of potassium.

## *What about the development of gout?*

Most authorities feel that gout and gouty arthritis are inherited diseases associated with an increase in the level of uric acid in the blood. The thiazide diuretics cause an increase in blood level of uric acid in 50 to 85 percent of patients. There is no doubt, therefore, that, if one has inherited that defect associated with gout, the thiazides may bring it to the surface and, indeed, cause gouty arthritis. It is essential, therefore, to monitor the level of uric acid in the blood just as we have to monitor glucose and potassium. If the symptoms of gout appear or if the uric acid level is over 10 mg%, drugs such as allopurinol (Zyloprin) or probenemid (Benemid) should be used. This does not mean, however, that the thiazides should be discontinued or that they are contraindicated in patients with gout.

## High blood pressure drugs and their side effects

The following list summarizes the current high blood pressure drugs available, with the generic names followed in parentheses by the registered trade names under which they are sold. Also included are the side effects that are sometimes produced, and what can be done to help eliminate those side effects.

### THIAZIDES AND RELATED DIURETICS

Thiazides and related diuretics (Diuril, Hydrodiuril, Esidrix, Orectic, Saluron, Naturetin, Naqua, Metahydrin, Enduron, Exna, Renese, Anhydron, Hygroton). *Side effects*: Decreased potassium levels with muscle cramps and gastrointestinal distress; to treat, take supplemental potassium or stop drug and use potassium-sparing drugs. Excess uric acid in the blood; to treat, use probenecid, allopurinol, or colchicine. Hypotension; to treat, decrease frequency and dose. Generalized aching; no good treatment.

### LOOP DIURETICS

Furosemide (Lasix). *Side effects*: Same as thiazides.
   Ethacrynic acid (Edecrin). *Side effects*: Same as thiazides.

### POTASSIUM-SPARING DIURETICS

Spironolactone (Aldactone). *Side effects*: Nausea, vomiting; to treat, take drugs after meals. Weakness, headache, or rash; to treat, decrease dosage. Enlargement of mammary glands in men; discontinue drug.

Triamterence (Dyrenium). *Side effects*: Same as spirono-lactone, except for mammary enlargement.

### RAUWOLFIA SERPENTINA

Reserpine (Serpasil, Sandril, Reserpoid, Raudixin, Rauwil-oid). *Side effects*: Nasal congestion; to treat, use nasal vasoconstrictor. Weight gain; use diuretics and stricter diet. Gastrointestinal bleeding; stop drug, switch to methyldopa. Lethargy, sluggishness; stop drug. Depression; stop drug. Nightmares; stop drug. Decreased libido; pray.

### METHYLDOPA (Aldomet)

*Side effects*: Drowsiness and dryness of mouth; symptoms usually diminish after first few weeks. Mood disturbances; stop drug. Slowed heartbeat; decrease dosage. Hemolytic anemia; watch with frequent blood tests.

### HYDRALAZINE (Apresoline)

*Side effects*: Headaches; to treat, add reserpine or take antihistamine medicine. Angina, rapid heartbeat, palpita-tions; treat with reserpine. Swelling of feet and ankles; treat with diuretics. General muscle pain; usually remits sponta-neously—if not, discontinue drug. Severe skin eruptions; discontinue drug.

### GUANETHIDINE (Ismelin)

*Side effects*: Dizziness, fainting; wear support stockings, get out of bed slowly, don't stand in one place for a long time, decrease dosage. Diarrhea; treat with atropine or other medicine. Fluid retention; treat with diuretics. Failure of ejaculation; sexual activity may be continued, don't worry about it, not harmful.

## *What about tranquilizers?*

Usually tranquilizer pills are not used unless stress is one of the chief causes of that particular person's high blood pressure. They should not be substituted for drugs that lower blood pressure. If a person really has severe anxiety, and can't do his job effectively because he is so upset, then tranquilizer pills may be effective.

### *Can I adjust my medication myself according to how I feel?*

Absolutely not! First, always remember that you cannot tell what your blood pressure is by the way you feel. Decreasing the number of pills could allow your pressure to reach dangerous heights. Increasing the pills could bring on undesirable side effects.

Blood pressure medicine is powerful stuff. It is great because it can save your life, but it should never be used except according to the directions of your physician. Just to show you the importance of sticking to his directions, advertising in medical journals even tells physicians: "Warn your patients not to deviate from instructions."

### *Can I ever stop taking them?*

Absolutely not! The treatment of high blood pressure is a lifetime affair. You can't stop taking your pills even though you feel great because the blood pressure may shoot right back up again and silently begin again to cause its killing damage.

### *Do the medicines cure the high blood pressure?*

Except for the kind that can be cured by surgery, at present no high blood pressure can be permanently cured. But it can be controlled. Simply by taking a pill a day, or maybe more, you can keep the blood pressure down to normal.

# 9

# *Designing a Personal Program*

High blood pressure can be even more dangerous than we have told you so far.

By itself it is bad enough as a threat to shortening your life. But it can be even more dangerous in conjunction with other risk factors like obesity and smoking. High blood pressure then becomes more lethal in promoting heart attacks and strokes.

It works this way. The main factors that seem to increase risk of heart attacks and strokes are high blood pressure, family history of heart attacks and strokes, smoking, high blood cholesterol, diabetes, obesity, and lack of exercise.

The greatest of these is high blood pressure. But add on one or two of the other risk factors and you have an explosive situation.

How important are these risk factors? If you have high blood pressure, they are the key to your health.

Consider these figures. If you are between ages thirty and fifty-nine and you have high blood pressure and *do not* have it treated, your chances of dying in the next ten years are twice as high as the chances of a person who doesn't have high blood pressure.

*If you have high blood pressure and also smoke cigarettes, or have high cholesterol,* your risk of dying in those ten years more than triples.

And if you have high blood pressure *and* smoke *and* have high cholesterol, the death rate is *five* times higher.

If you have high blood pressure and smoke, your chances of having a *stroke* are sixteen times higher!

The risks don't just add on. They *multiply*. And if you have a heart attack, they make the heart attack worse. If you have a stroke, it is more deadly. And if you have one stroke or heart attack, they make it more likely you will have a second.

Whether you have high blood pressure or not, controlling these other factors will decrease your risk of heart disease and stroke and may help you avoid an early death.

If you do have high blood pressure, controlling the other factors can be vital and life-saving.

If you have high blood pressure, there is a side advantage, too. If you control these other risk factors, it often *reduces* your blood pressure as well as reducing risk of heart attack and stroke. And almost always your doctor then can reduce the amount of medicine you need to take. The lower the dosage, the fewer the side effects. One patient, Bill L., lost weight until he was trim, gave up smoking, and watched his diet carefully. He was able to lower his blood pressure so much he was able to stop taking his medication. In most cases, the medicine can be reduced, but not stopped; and even this, of course, should only be done under the careful guidance of your physician.

In this chapter we will help you discover exactly what your particular risk factors are and will advise you on planning a specific program to combat these factors.

### *Is there scientific evidence for these added dangers?*

Yes. Many studies have shown that men with high blood pressure had a higher mortality rate than men with normal pressures. When they were also overweight, the mortality rate doubled.

A study of teen-age college students showed that those with a systolic pressure of 130 or higher had a death rate 60 percent higher in the next decades than those with lower pressures, and a systolic pressure of 130 is considered *"normal."* If they were also in the habit of smoking ten or more cigarettes daily, their risk of early death was doubled.

The correlations were probably shown most dramatically in the ten-year study of the men in Chicago working at the People's Gas Company. The death rate for a man aged forty to fifty-nine with no risk factors was forty-four deaths per one thousand. If he had high blood pressure, the death rate tripled to 137 per one thousand. If he had high blood pressure and high cholesterol and smoked, his death rate was five times higher, or 220 deaths per one thousand.

Here is a table that shows all their results.

---

RELATIONSHIP BETWEEN BLOOD PRESSURE, OTHER RISK FACTORS, AND TEN-YEAR MORTALITY FROM ALL CAUSES.

| *1958 risk-factor status* | *Ten-year death rate per one thousand* |
|---|---|
| None of four factors high | 44 |
| Hypertension—only one of four factors | 137 |
| Hypercholesterolemia, heavy cigarette smoking, rapid heart rate— any one only—without hypertension | 79 |
| Hypercholesterolemia, heavy cigarette smoking, rapid heart rate— any one only—with hypertension | 158 |

Hypercholesterolemia, heavy cigarette
smoking, rapid heart rate—
any two or all three—without hypertension      170

Hypercholesterolemia, heavy cigarette
smoking, rapid heart rate—
any two or all three—with hypertension       220

### *Do many people have these combinations of factors?*

Too many.

About one in four middle-aged men and women have an elevated serum cholesterol level of 260 mg. and higher. About one out of three men and women are 20 percent or more above optimum weight. Approximately one in six men smokes over twenty cigarettes a day.

At ages fifty-five to sixty-four the numbers of people with elevated serum cholesterol levels and excess weight are even higher.

When you figure how many people also have high blood pressure, it is no wonder heart disease and stroke have become the biggest killers of this century.

### *Do these other risk factors* cause *high blood pressure?*

They don't actually cause the high blood pressure, but they do add to the complications and increase your chances of dying prematurely or being seriously crippled in your everyday living.

The risk factors will also help determine how serious your complications may be. They may make the difference between whether you have only chest pains or a full-blown heart attack; or if you do have a heart attack or stroke, whether you live or die.

## *What can be done about these factors?*

There is nothing you can do about a family history of heart attack and stroke, but there is much you can do about the other risk factors. You can help prevent strokes, heart disease, and the other serious complications that can result from hypertension by attacking on six major fronts.

1. You can determine whether you have high blood pressure and, if so, take medicines for it.

2. You can stop smoking cigarettes.

3. You can change to a diet lower in cholesterols, fats, and sugars, and, if you have high pressure, cut down on salt.

4. If you are fat, you can lose weight.

5. You can begin regular habits of moderate exercise.

6. You can try to relax more if you tend to over-react to stress.

## *If I take high blood pressure medicine, do I need to do these other things?*

For a really comprehensive and effective approach you should do your best to work on all of them. Life is a gamble for sure, but the smart person plays as many odds in his favor as he can for a better and longer life.

Working on some of the risk factors will directly lower your blood pressure. With others, we are not sure of their effect on the blood pressure, but we know they are an added risk for a stroke and heart disease and therefore worth working on. At least, it will help your general health and sense of well-being.

## *Special risk factors for women*

Women have two additional risk factors: premature menopause—whether natural or as a result of removal of the ovaries—and the use of contraceptives.

We will discuss these further in a later chapter.

## *Figuring your own risk profile*

We've been talking a lot about the statistics of other people's health. Now let's figure out exactly what your own personal risk profile is, what your chances are of having a stroke or heart attack.

Score yourself right now, or if you do not know all the medical facts, such as serum cholesterol levels, wait until you can get them from your doctor.

1. What is your diastolic (lower number) blood pressure? *1 point if it is 85 or 100, and 2 points if it is over 100.*

2. Are you overweight? *1 point if you are more than thirty pounds over the standard weight for your height.*

3. Do you smoke? *If so, 1 point. For two packs a day, 2 points.*

4. Do you regularly exercise or are you more sedentary? *If sedentary, 1 point.*

5. Do you or your parents or your family have diabetes? *If someone in your family, 1 point; if you have it, 2 points.*

6. Have your parents or any brothers or sisters had a heart attack or stroke before age sixty? *If yes, 1 point.*

7. Do you have an elevated serum cholesterol value? *If mildly elevated cholesterol (210 to 250 mg. percent), 1 point. If high (over 250), 2 points.*

8. Was your last electrocardiogram normal or abnormal? *If the doctor said there were some abnormalities in your EKG, 1 point.*

Add up your risk points. The total gives your personal risk profile.

If your points total 0–2, you are at low risk of having a heart attack or stroke. If you scored 3–5 points, you have a moderate risk. If you have 6–12 points, you are under very high risk.

## *Working up your own needs*

Look over the questions again, and see what risk factors pertain to you. Then determine which ones are fixable. For example, one of your parents having had a heart attack at a young age is a factor you cannot change. High blood pressure or diabetes you *can* control by taking medicines. Then, knowing yourself, knowing how high or low your personal risk is, knowing how much you really do or don't want to design a program to fight this risk, determine what factors you are willing to change. They really make a difference in your life enjoyment and life expectancy, both for the next few years and for the long-term future.

Don't say you're too busy. Don't say, "It won't happen to me." Don't wait till you get a heart attack or stroke to get the message.

Now that you know your needs, the knowledge needs to be translated into action. And that's what the next four chapters are for—to tell you exactly how you can alter your diet, stop smoking, get beneficial exercise and cut down stress.

# 10

# Reducing Risks by What You Eat

Every time you sit down at the table, what you reach for and how much of it you reach for helps determine what your chances are of having a long healthy life, or of dying early from a heart attack or stroke.

There are three areas in which you can eat yourself to death—or to health. One is in the number of calories you eat and whether you become overweight from too many of them. Another is the amount and kinds of fats you eat, and whether they give you high cholesterol levels. A third—important if you have high blood pressure—is the amount of salt you eat with your food.

Obesity, high cholesterol, and salt have all been blamed as villains in adding to the problems of high blood pressure, adding to the risks of heart attack, stroke, and kidney disease.

Take obesity, for example. In one day, the heart of an average-sized adult pumps the equivalent of four thousand gallons of blood. Each pound of fat forces the heart to pump that blood through 200 more miles of blood vessels. Carrying around just fifteen pounds of excess weight means your heart has to pump blood an extra three thousand miles, the width of the United States from coast to coast!

People who are overweight have high blood pressure much more frequently than those who are not overweight. And as you go from young adulthood to middle age, the more weight you gain, the greater is the tendency to high blood pressure.

One study showed that women who were severely overweight had three times more high blood pressure than women who were not overweight.

But being overweight does not *cause* high blood pressure. Fat people can have normal pressure, and skinny people can have high pressure.

At middle age, the man who is overweight is two to three times more susceptible to coronary heart disease than the man of normal weight. John T., who has gained 20 percent more weight since he was a young man, is at least twice as prone to a heart attack as Oliver J., who stays lean.

As a matter of fact, John has high blood pressure in addition to being overweight, which makes his risk of premature heart attack about four times the normal risk.

Being overweight is so detrimental to your health that physicians at the Metropolitan Life Insurance Company say you can roughly calculate how long you will live by taking a single test. Measure your chest. Then measure your waist. For every inch your waist exceeds your chest, they say, take two years off your normal life expectancy. Their statistics show that policyholders who were 30 percent or more overweight had a mortality rate 35 percent higher than those policyholders who weighed less.

And dropping excess pounds can save you money on your life insurance policy, too. Life insurance companies for many years have asked a higher premium from the obese man, reducing it when the policyholder brought his weight down, because his risks of dying early have been reduced.

### *Does losing weight help control high blood pressure?*

There's some evidence that if fat people reduce, their blood pressure does go down, but why is not known.

Some people believe it is getting rid of the excess pounds itself that does the trick. Others believe that the benefit comes from the fact that getting rid of weight also gets rid of excess salt.

In Framingham, of those people with high blood pressure who were able to lose weight, about 60 percent had their pressure drop.

### *If I follow a diet plan, can I give up blood pressure pills?*

The major problem with diet plans is that most people don't stick to them. The result is their weight goes up and down, up and down, in what nutritionists call the yoyo effect.

The truth is that if you get your weight down and keep it down, the chances are your blood pressure will drop considerably. But you must *keep* the weight down. John with his weight problem found his eating so important and dieting such a problem, that it was easier and more reliable for him simply to take a pill a day for high blood pressure. Others find dieting not such a problem once they develop new eating habits, and they are overjoyed to be able to stop taking pills or to be able to take smaller dosages. As we have said before, and it cannot be said too often, changes in your medicines should only be made on your doctor's instructions.

Weight loss is especially effective in people with only slightly elevated pressures, under 100 mm Hg. diastolic, so slight that the doctor hesitates to start them on blood pressure medicines, and yet the pressure is above normal.

This was the case with Sally R. Losing weight brought her pressure completely down to normal. You still must keep in touch with your doctor, however, because you never know if or when it's going to creep back up.

### Fat children

We used to say, "A fat baby is a healthy baby."

Perhaps it's a legacy from the times when many people were too poor to feed their children well, and the chubbier youngsters were better able to fight off diseases.

But medical thinking now is trying to torpedo this belief—because too often the fat baby and the fat child grow up to be the fat adult. Children are inclined to adopt their parents' eating habits, whether good or bad.

A recent study from Georgia, which followed children with slightly elevated blood pressure, demonstrated that those who were overweight in addition to having high blood pressure were the ones who developed subsequent heart damage or stroke.

### What is the best way to lose weight?

Begin slowly, with smaller portions of what you ordinarily eat. Cut down especially on high-calorie foods. Remember that extra calories build into excess pounds.

### Will a good "crash diet" do it more quickly?

There are lots of crash diets, and "new" ones keep popping up. Almost all share one common flaw—they ask you to do something quite different from your present eating habits. Any one of them may melt off pounds quickly; the trouble lies in trying to stick with it. Because their requirements are too extreme, you tend to slip back to your old eating habits, and sooner or later, the calories and pounds climb back aboard again.

It took you some time to gain those pounds. Taking time to get them off again—slowly but steadily—is the best way to drop them.

## What about diet pills?

Although several weight-reducing pills are now available and approved by the Food and Drug Administration, their effects seem short-lived and their side effects limit their usefulness. A large number of people say the pills cause diarrhea and other gastrointestinal upsets, or cause excitability and disturb sleep.

It is best to lose weight without pills.

## Helpful hints to losing weight

If you need to lose weight, the following suggestions should help you.

Purchase a small calorie-counting book—and carry it with you. When you reach for food, consult your guide and select only low-calorie foods.

Keep a ready supply of low-calorie snacks handy at all times.

No second helpings.

Remove high-calorie foods from your diet. Try eating bread without butter. On baked potato, instead of butter, use a dab of sour cream. Replace the sugar in your coffee with an artificial sweetener. Eat only one dessert a day. Then eat fresh fruit or a small amount of sweet food to satisfy a craving for a richer dessert. Beware of cocktails and beers, both high in calories.

Divide portions of food. Instead of a whole Danish for

breakfast and another later, divide it, eating half for breakfast and the other half later at half the calories.

Get plenty of exercise—a good brisk walk around the block at lunch and before and after dinner. As a matter of fact, walk whenever you can. The daily exercise will not only help burn up calories, but will also improve your circulation and muscle tone.

Don't take calories to bed with you. Calories are used up in two to three hours after you consume them. If not used up within that time, they are not used at all. Therefore, it's poor practice to eat before going to bed. The secret of losing weight, in addition to reducing calories, is to eat three meals regularly—more at breakfast and lunch, a smaller than normal amount at dinner, and nothing after dinner. In this way your normal activities during the day will burn up the calories you consume.

### Behavioral control

Many people have found help from the principles of behavioral control. They find ways to enhance the positive aspects of dieting and they set up negative thoughts against the foods they want to avoid. They work at it consciously at first, and soon the newly set up behavior patterns become automatic and habitual.

If it works for you, fine. We're not against anything that works.

One successful dieter took "before" photographs in a bathing suit that showed his bulging belly and double chins. He pasted copies of the photo on the kitchen door and on the refrigerator as a constant reminder of how far he had come.

Another dieter closed his eyes every time he went through a cafeteria line or grocery store and pictured himself lying in a coffin with a lily in his hand so he would not reach for fattening foods. Another pictures a skull and crossbones painted on high-calorie foods.

Some dieters put small portions on tiny plates, desserts in frappé glasses to make them look bigger. Or they cut one slice of bread into four portions so it seems as if they are getting more.

One man has a basket in his refrigerator marked "Survival Kit" and keeps it stocked with celery and carrot sticks, oranges, radishes, low-cal soda, and other low-calorie items for those times when he feels hungry enough to eat everything in sight.

Make your meals attractive and interesting. *Low calorie* doesn't have to mean boring. Experiment with new recipes, foreign or exotic dishes, marinating sauces, herbs, and spices.

When you eat out, go to a seafood restaurant, where you can eat great-tasting fish dishes with little calorie input. Order à la carte, so you won't feel like you're wasting money by passing up the side dishes.

Accentuate the positive. Reward yourself for good behavior. When you've lost the first five pounds, celebrate with flowers on the table. For the next five, have candlelight and silver or a trip to the theater. For a bigger weight loss, buy yourself something terrific.

### *Figuring your own calorie formula*

Calories are the units of energy found in all foods. Excess is stored as fat. Take in more than you use up, and you put on weight. It's that simple. So, to lose weight you have to figure out your formula of intake and output.

Most people, leading moderately active lives, use about 15 calories per pound to maintain their weight. So if you want to stay at 150 pounds, $15 \times 150 = 2,250$, the maximum number of calories you can consume in one day.

According to the Council on Foods and Nutrition of the American Medical Association, to *lose* one pound a week, you need to consume 500 fewer calories per day. So to lose one pound a week you need to subtract 500 calories from your calorie maintenance level. If you want to lose two pounds per week then you must subtract 1,000 calories per day.

To find your formula, write down your desired weight. (Ask your doctor, or see weight chart.) Multiply it by 15. From the total, if you want to lose one pound per week, subtract 500. If you want to lose two pounds per week, subtract 1,000. This will give you the maximum number of calories you can have in a day.

Write the number down so you can refer to it in the future.

Or another method is to eat everything you` would ordinarily eat over a three-day period, writing down every peanut and canapé. Then look at a calorie list—you can get one at any drugstore—and total up your average daily calorie intake. Try to plan your eating so you take in only about half that amount of calories, and you will be sure to lose some weight.

You might also find it helpful to make a chart to keep a record of your weight. Write down the weight you would really like to be. Then mark your weight down on the chart each week so you can see your progress as you follow your weight reducing plan.

### Weight chart

Locate your height on this chart to find your recommended weight. The figures are for men and women over age twenty-five with a medium frame. If you have a small body frame, your ideal weight would be 5 to 10 pounds less. If you have a large frame, it could be 8 to 14 pounds more.

These body weights, prepared by the Metropolitan Life

Insurance Company, have been observed to be associated with the lowest mortality rate.

| MEN | | | WOMEN | | |
|---|---|---|---|---|---|
| Height | | Medium | Height | | Medium |
| Feet | Inches | Frame | Feet | Inches | Frame |
| 5 | 2 | 118–129 | 4 | 10 | 96–107 |
| 5 | 3 | 121–133 | 4 | 11 | 98–110 |
| 5 | 4 | 124–136 | 5 | 0 | 101–113 |
| 5 | 5 | 127–139 | 5 | 1 | 104–116 |
| 5 | 6 | 130–143 | 5 | 2 | 107–119 |
| 5 | 7 | 134–147 | 5 | 3 | 110–122 |
| 5 | 8 | 138–152 | 5 | 4 | 113–126 |
| 5 | 9 | 142–156 | 5 | 5 | 116–130 |
| 5 | 10 | 146–160 | 5 | 6 | 120–135 |
| 5 | 11 | 150–165 | 5 | 7 | 124–139 |
| 6 | 0 | 154–170 | 5 | 8 | 128–143 |
| 6 | 1 | 158–175 | 5 | 9 | 132–147 |
| 6 | 2 | 162–180 | 5 | 10 | 136–151 |
| 6 | 3 | 167–185 | 5 | 11 | 140–155 |
| 6 | 4 | 172–190 | 6 | 0 | 144–159 |

## *What about cholesterol and fats?*

High blood cholesterol greatly increases the chances of premature death. Combined with high blood pressure, as noted earlier, it multiplies those chances even more.

Cholesterol is a waxy material that forms part of the fatty deposits that can plug up vital arteries to bring on heart attacks or strokes.

The American Heart Association and others have called for modification of our diets, to reduce consumption of saturated (animal and dairy) fats and to reduce consumption of foods containing cholesterol.

These diet changes have been shown to reduce blood cholesterol levels and fatty deposits in artery channels, but for a long time it was not fully proved that the changes actually prevented strokes and heart attacks, and there was a great deal of controversy.

Now the evidence is coming in that these diet changes do decrease the occurrence of heart disease and stroke. According to a recent joint statement by the Food and Nutrition Board, National Academy of Sciences, and the Council on Foods and Nutrition of the American Medical Association, "The evidence now available is sufficient to discourage further temporizing with this major national health problem."

### *How common is high cholesterol in the blood?*

Too common.

Some years ago doctors performing autopsies on young American soldiers discovered that many of them already had signs of the beginnings of atherosclerosis in their coronary arteries. Their average age was twenty-two! Other researchers have found similar fatty deposits in the arteries of teenagers and even children.

For example, fifteen-year-old boys in Boston were found to have serum cholesterol levels similar to men in their forties and fifties in areas of the world where coronary heart disease is rare.

In Louisiana, Dr. Gerald S. Berenson and colleagues found three-year-old children with serum cholesterol levels already as high as those of adults.

In a study in Arizona, Drs. Glenn Friedman and Stanley J. Goldberg found that 10 to 35 percent of children studied there had excess cholesterol in their blood. Some were not even a year old.

The earlier you start on a proper diet the better for health.

In Muscatine, Iowa, where such high-risk children were found, concerned people launched a special diet program to try to change these factors. They altered the school's lunch program to provide skim milk, margarine, and low-cholesterol foods. Dieticians instructed the mothers in home meal planning. Also, whenever they found a child who had high blood fat they checked the family. By instructing them on a 20 percent fat, 100-milligram cholesterol diet, they were able to lower the cholesterol of the affected members by 60 percent.

### *Exactly what is cholesterol?*

It is a fatty chemical produced in the liver. It also occurs in such foods as butter, eggs, cheese, and animal fats. In the body it helps transport fat through the bloodstream and also is important in the production of bile and certain hormones. The higher the levels of cholesterol, the higher the risk of dying prematurely.

### *What is atherosclerosis?*

It is a disease characterized by deposits of cholesterol and fatty substances called lipoproteins on interior walls of arteries. According to the National Center for Health Statistics, almost half of all U.S. deaths last year were traceable to atherosclerosis.

### *What are saturated and unsaturated fats?*

Saturated fats are fats that harden at room temperature. They tend to raise the level of cholesterol in the blood. They are found in most meat, in butter, cream, and whole milk, in some cheeses, in many solid and hydrogenated shortenings, and in coconut oil, cocoa butter, and palm oil.

Polyunsaturated fats, which are recommended, are usually liquid oils of vegetable origin. Oils such as corn, cottonseed, safflower, sesame seed, soybean, and sunflower seed are high in polyunsaturated fat. They tend to lower the level of cholesterol in the blood by helping the body to eliminate the excess.

Hydrogenation changes liquid fats to solid fats. Completely hydrogenated (hardened) oils resemble saturated fats and should be avoided or used in moderation; but margarines and shortenings containing partially hydrogenated oils also contain acceptable amounts of polyunsaturates.

### *Does lowering fat and cholesterol intake do anything to blood pressure?*

What is believed to be the first research data to show that blood pressure can be lowered by reducing the level of fat in an otherwise normal diet was reported this year at a meeting of the American Heart Association by Dr. James M. Iacono, a nutritionist with the U.S. Department of Agriculture.

The study was conducted jointly by the USDA and Georgetown University School of Medicine.

The percentage of calories provided by fats in typical U.S. diets is in the 40 to 45 percent range. When fat levels were dropped below this range in volunteers, blood pressures were decreased significantly and promptly, Dr. Iacono said.

### *Keeping cholesterol down*

To achieve a low blood cholesterol level, the rules are fairly simple.

Eat fewer foods high in saturated fats, that is, the hard fats. Eat fewer foods high in cholesterol, such as the yolk of eggs. And put more emphasis on foods high in polyunsaturated fats, generally those of vegetable origin.

Under this basic plan, you would use safflower, corn, cottonseed, or soy oil for cooking; cut down on eggs, and egg yolk; serve more veal, fish and chicken, and trim the excess fat off beef, pork and lamb; and replace butter with a polyunsaturated margarine.

You can still eat well while doing this, like a gourmet in fact. The recently published *American Heart Association Cookbook* contains five hundred great recipes.

Other books with recipes for a low-cholesterol *haute cuisine: 1973 Metropolitan Cookbook*, available free from Metropolitan Life Insurance Company, 1 Madison Ave., New York, N.Y. 10010; *Dietary Control of Cholesterol*, available from Fleishmann's Margarines, 625 Madison Ave., New York, N.Y. 10022; and *A Way of Life: Planned Low-Fat Cholesterol Recipes*, available from the DeKalb County Medical Society, 755 Columbus Dr., Decatur, Ga. 30030.

### *Cholesterol contents of common foods*

## MEAT, FISH AND EGGS
### (3-ounce [85 gm] serving)

| | Cholesterol (mg) |
|---|---|
| Liver (cooked) | 372 |
| Egg (1 large—50 gm) | 252 |
| Shrimp (canned, drained solids) | 128 |
| Veal (cooked) | 86 |
| Lamb (cooked) | 83 |
| Beef (cooked) | 80 |
| Pork (cooked) | 76 |
| Chicken (cooked) | 74 |
| Lobster (meat only—cooked) | 72 |

| | |
|---|---|
| Fish (raw) | 43–60 |
| Oysters (meat only—raw) | 43 |
| Clams (meat only—raw) | 43 |

## DAIRY FOODS

| | |
|---|---|
| Whole milk (8-oz. glass) | 34 |
| American cheese (1 oz.) | 28 |
| Ice cream (½ cup) | 27–49 |
| Gouda cheese (1 oz.) | 21 |
| Heavy whipping cream (1 tbsp.) | 20 |
| Yogurt (1 cup) | 17 |
| Cottage cheese (½ cup) | 12–24 |
| Butter (1 tsp.) | 12 |
| Half and Half (1 tbsp.) | 6 |
| Skim milk (8-oz. glass) | 5 |

## *The Prudent Diet*

Several groups, including the American Heart Association, have now endorsed a diet called the Prudent Diet, which takes into account all the latest findings about the role diet plays in high blood pressure and heart disease.

Principles of the Prudent Diet are:

Reduced calories.

Reduced fat.

Increased polyunsaturates.

Reduced cholesterol.

Adjusted carbohydrate. (Deriving carbohydrates from grain, fruits and vegetables instead of sugars.)

Reduced salt intake.

Stabilized protein intake. (Proteins should contribute 12 percent to 15 percent of each day's calories.)

## *Putting the Prudent Diet to work*

If you would like to use the recommended Prudent Diet to improve your health and your family's, follow these guidelines. They are designed for the typical American family.

Cut calories by cutting down on desserts, pastries, fat meats, snack foods, beer, sweet wines, hard liquors, and soft drinks sweetened with sugar.

Cut fats by restricting fatty foods and allowing only two tablespoons of vegetable oil a day for salad dressings, cooking, and baking. To be avoided: butter, lard, hard cooking fats, margarines high in saturated fats, and cream substitutes.

Main dishes, for lunch or dinner, should include fish and poultry several times a week.

Choose lean cuts of meat, trim visible fat, and discard the fat that cooks out of the meat. Avoid deep fat frying; use baking, boiling, broiling, roasting, stewing. Instead of butter and solid cooking fats, use liquid vegetable oils and margarines. Avoid fatty meats such as bacon, frankfurters, corned beef, pastrami, salami, and sausage. No gravies.

No more than three eggs a week for adults, seven for children.

Only skim or low-fat milk for adults, limited to a pint a day. Children may have a pint of whole milk daily, but any more than that should be low-fat or skimmed.

Cottage, pot, and farmer cheese are low in fat and high in protein and may be used often. To be avoided: butter, sweet cream, sour cream, cream cheese, ice cream. Total of such cheeses as cheddar, American, Swiss, and Camembert should be less than four ounces a week.

Dark-green, leafy, and deep-yellow vegetables should be eaten at least four times a week. Others, including potatoes, can be used freely.

At least one high-vitamin-C fruit (orange, tomato, grapefruit, or cantaloupe) should be served daily, and unsweetened fruits as desired.

Whole-grain or enriched bread, or cereal, may be used with every meal. Nuts, seeds, and beans are nutritionally valuable.

### *What about alcohol and coffee?*

The immediate effect of alcohol ingestion is to raise the blood pressure slightly. When the effect of alcohol wears off the blood pressure returns to its former level.

As a matter of fact, social drinking—even as much as six drinks a day—is associated with a lower-than-normal risk of a heart attack.

However, there is increased high blood pressure in severe chronic alcoholics, and *heavy* drinking is associated with a higher risk of heart attack and stroke. So social drinking is okay for the person with high blood pressure, but excess use of alcohol is bad. And we've recently learned that even social drinking temporarily reduces work capacity or exercise tolerance if a person has a damaged heart.

Coffee and tea also produce a temporary rise in blood pressure, but the increase disappears after the effects of the caffeine have worn off.

In a study in California there was no correlation found between coffee drinking and heart attacks. But another international study suggested that people drinking more than five cups per day have about twice as great a risk of a heart attack as people drinking no coffee at all.

One thing that seems to make coffee drinking dangerous is that heavy coffee drinkers are usually heavy cigarette smokers.

Cigarette smoking, we know, increases the likelihood of a heart attack.

## Salt and high blood pressure

It is generally agreed that there definitely is some tie-in between salt and high blood pressure. How closely the two are related and how important it is to not use salt if you have high blood pressure is where the arguments begin.

Salt is really sodium chloride. And what we are talking about is the sodium in the salt, the damaging part.

Much of the evidence for the importance of salt or sodium in high blood pressure comes from the work of Dr. Lewis K. Dahl of Brookhaven National Laboratory in Upton, New York.

Dr. Dahl and his colleagues compared salt intake and high blood pressure in six widely differing populations of the world: Americans, Alaskan Eskimos, Marshall Islanders, northern and southern Japanese, and Bantus of South Africa. They found a dramatic correlation between average daily salt intake and hypertension. Eskimos, for example, eat almost no salt, and have extremely low rates of hypertension—1 to 2 percent. In northern Japan the daily intake of salt ranges from forty to fifty grams, and almost 50 percent of the people have hypertension!

In the Solomon Islands in the South Pacific, Dr. Lot Page studied eight different groups of native islanders, some living by the sea, some in the picturesque high mountains, some fishermen, some settled farmers, and some "slash-and-burn" farmers who clear land, grow crops, and move on after a season.

Of the eight groups, he found six that had no high blood pressure and no coronary vascular disease. Two groups had a rise in blood pressure and cholesterol with age.

The differences? The islanders with high blood pressure used salt in their diet. The others did not. And the highest blood pressure was in the tribe that had the highest salt intake.

Dr. Dahl also studied the effects of salt on some forty-five thousand laboratory rats. (Researchers made a tiny donut-shaped blood pressure cuff and measured blood pressure in the tail.) The results indicated that salt definitely caused high blood pressure in them. When a colony of rats was fed a high-salt diet, in about 2 to 5 percent "the blood pressure took off like a rocket," Dr. Dahl says, "and these died with malignant hypertension in two to three months." In about 25 percent of the colony the blood pressure remained normal. About 70 percent or so developed varying in-between degrees of hypertension.

Dahl was able to breed the rats into two strains—one that was resistant to salt and one that always got high blood pressure from a high salt diet.

Dr. Dahl believes that a predisposition to the disease plus salt or other factors is what gives high blood pressure in both rats and man. Whether salt plays a role in causing high blood pressure in any one person depends on his genetic makeup plus how much salt he eats.

The amount of potassium and calcium you take in may be important, too. Eating more of these seems to protect somewhat against sodium.

### What's the theory about salt?

Salt is well known to be involved in body systems that maintain blood pressure. It promotes retention of water in the body, and this adds to the volume of blood that needs to be pumped around. It also seems to affect the diameter of the arterioles.

### How much sodium should we use?

The estimated daily sodium requirement is only one-half to one gram. Most Americans consume five to twenty times that amount, for a daily average of fourteen grams (half an ounce). Probably half of this is added during cooking or at the table.

Some people, however, use up to 25 grams a day, almost a full ounce. And many people have a tendency over the years to keep increasing their sodium intake, developing a taste for saltier and saltier foods.

### *Does cutting down on salt reduce blood pressure?*

Blood pressures do come down when people eat a diet containing practically no salt. One diet effective in doing this was the rice and fruit diet, prescribed some years ago, that was even effective in controlling people with malignant hypertension. Its major value was the fact that it contained less than two hundred milligrams of sodium. The diet itself was very bland and boring to try to stick with.

There is some evidence that the reason weight loss reduces blood pressure is that, as food intake is cut down, salt intake is reduced. Some researchers found that the person losing weight does not get lower pressure if his salt intake is kept high. However, more research needs to be done in this area.

### *What is the salt reduction necessary to affect blood pressure?*

A reduction from two hundred to five hundred milligrams of sodium (five hundred milligrams equals half a gram) daily, most doctors say. But this is difficult to achieve, since sodium is in so many foods. For example, one glass of milk supplies two hundred milligrams of sodium. (Skim milk has an even higher content of sodium than whole milk. So you shouldn't drink any milk at all if you are on a sodium-restricted diet.)

However, in Evans County, Georgia, a group of patients with high blood pressure was treated with a relatively low sodium diet (three grams per day), and blood pressure levels decreased. When many of those on drug treatment also went on a weight-reducing and low-salt diet, many were able to give up their blood pressure medication.

Usually you cannot tell how successful a low-sodium diet will be until you have followed it for several months.

Diuretic pills, the major pills used to treat high blood pressure, act by eliminating salt and water from your body by increasing kidney action.

Some specialists say if you take your blood pressure pills, you don't have to worry about salt. Others think, however, that taking in large amounts of salt a day counteracts a good deal of the beneficial effect of the drugs. They believe that a reduction in salt intake makes it easier for the drugs to work. The amount of medication often can be reduced if salt intake is reduced.

Some patients consume such large quantities of salt that average doses of diuretics cannot overcome it, and consequently their hypertension may not respond readily to the usual doses of medicine. When this occurs, salt in the diet definitely needs to be cut back.

The opinion held by most doctors is: if you take your pills regularly, you need not suffer through a completely salt-free diet, but you should use moderation in salt, cutting back as much as you can.

Your doctor, by the way, can check your sodium levels with a simple urine test.

### Salt in prepared foods

Some doctors also favor taking salt out of prepared baby foods, because babies don't need it, and it may pave the way for future high blood pressure. This is in line with one theory that a child's kidney may be especially sensitive to damage from excess salt. The American Academy of Pediatrics reports that dietary intake of salt by infants sometimes exceeds minimum requirements by four to six times. Their Committee on Nutrition recommends restraint of the use of salt by food processors and urges labeling concerning the amount of salt added to processed foods.

### Should I throw away my salt shaker?

Not necessarily, but use it sparingly. You may get five to ten grams of sodium from it daily if you are heavy-handed.

Cutting your consumption to two grams a day will help lower high blood pressure.

The American Heart Association recommends moderation in salt intake for everyone, whether they have high blood pressure or not.

### What is a low-sodium diet?

If you eat foods in a natural state, and avoid milk or milk protein, you can consider yourself on a low-salt diet. Lobster and certain seafoods are okay, but canned foods, which have been salted, are out.

Three major rules to reduce salt intake are:

Never add salt in preparation of food, or at the table.

Remember that milk and milk products are high in salt content.

Avoid canned or frozen foods, because sodium is used in canning, except in fruits and fruit juices, and even then check the label for salt content. A single serving of frozen lima beans, for example, has two hundred times more sodium than the same portion of fresh limas.

### Foods to avoid

If you are on a low-salt diet, you should avoid the following high-salt foods.

Salty or smoked meat such as: bacon, bologna, chipped or corned beef, frankfurters, ham, lunch meats, salt pork, sausage, smoked tongue

Salty or smoked fish such as: anchovies, caviar, salted and dried cod, herring, sardines

Processed cheese (unless it is low-sodium dietetic), cheese spreads, or any cheese such as Roquefort, Camembert, or Gorgonzola

Mustard, prepared

Onion salt

Relishes

Cooking wine

Worcestershire sauce

Commercial bouillon

Catsup

Celery salt

Chili sauce

Garlic salt

Meat extracts, sauces, and tenderizers (if not low-sodium dietetic)

Salted nuts

Olives

Potato chips, pretzels, salted popcorn or other heavily salted snack foods

Sauerkraut, pickles, or other vegetables prepared in brine or heavily salted

Breads and rolls with salt toppings

### Hints for the person on a low-sodium diet

• Several low-salt products are now on the market. Look for low-salt bread, low-salt soup, low-sodium milk. There is even a salt with less sodium.

• Also, pure coarse salt (the kind served in a salt mill, sometimes known as kosher salt) is saltier in taste than free-running shaker salt, so you get more taste from less salt.

• Don't use snuff or chew tobacco. They contain a lot of salt and may be responsible, some doctors think, for some of the high blood pressure in the southeast part of the United States.

• Don't eat licorice. It causes marked retention of salt and water in the body.

• Stay away from soul food that is high in salt. Dr. Emery Rann, president of the predominantly black National Medical Association, believes the high salt use of blacks is a major factor in their higher rate of high blood pressure.

• Fresh fish is sometimes packed in salt water. Rinse it before cooking.

• Stay away from foods that contain large amounts of sodium chloride, monosodium glutamate, sodium bicarbonate (baking soda) or brine (salt water used for pickling and preserving).

• Don't add salt or monosodium glutamate to food when you cook.

• Baking soda may be used in baking, but not as a remedy for indigestion or in cooking vegetables.

• Keep away from foods cured with salt (ham) or kept in brine (pickles, olives).

• Canned soup or stew may be too salty; for example, a ten-ounce can may easily contain twenty-two hundred to nine thousand milligrams of sodium.

Ask your doctor, your heart association, or health department about the sodium in your local water supply. Depending on its source, water may contain as little as one milligram or more than fifteen hundred milligrams of sodium per quart. Home installed water softeners should not be used as they usually add sodium to the water in the softening process.

Some medicines contain enough sodium to interfere with your diet. Always check with your doctor before you use any unprescribed medicine, even a headache remedy. Medicines that may contain sodium: alkalizers for indigestion (such as bicarbonate of soda, rhubarb and soda), antibiotics, cough medicines, laxatives, pain relievers, sedatives.

Toothpastes, tooth powders, and mouthwashes may also contain large amounts of sodium. Rinse your mouth well after using them.

## *What about using a salt substitute?*

A salt substitute may be used only when your doctor has recommended a specific kind. Some salt substitutes contain sodium and others are harmful to persons with certain diseases. Play safe and ask your doctor what kind of salt substitute, if any, you may use. The same goes for low-sodium meat tenderizers. None of them is very tasty anyway.

## *What can I do to keep food from tasting flat?*

There are many other seasonings that will keep your meals interesting. Here are some flavor ideas used by chefs in the world's best restaurants:

Beef: bay leaf, dry mustard, green pepper, grape jelly, sage, marjoram, mushrooms, nutmeg, onion, pepper, thyme

Chicken: cranberries, mushrooms, paprika, parsley, poultry seasoning, thyme, sage

Lamb: curry, garlic, mint, pineapple, rosemary

Pork: apples, applesauce, garlic, onion, sage

Veal: apricots, bay leaf, curry, currant jelly, ginger, marjoram, oregano, lemon juice

Fish: bay leaf, curry, dry mustard, green pepper, lemon juice, marjoram, mushrooms, paprika

EGGS: curry, dry mustard, green pepper, jelly, mushrooms, onion, paprika, parsley, tomato
ASPARAGUS: lemon juice
CORN: green pepper, tomato
GREEN BEANS: marjoram, lemon juice, nutmeg, dill seed, sugar, onion, unsalted French dressing
PEAS: onion, mint, mushrooms, parsley, green pepper
POTATOES: onion, mace, green pepper, parsley
SQUASH: ginger, mace, onion
TOMATOES: basil, marjoram, onion, celery, sugar

## What are dietetic foods?

Dietetic foods are those prepared for specific diets—diets restricted in sugar and starch, sodium, or fat, for example. The label must carry an exact statement of the contents. On dietetic foods prepared specifically for sodium-restricted diets, the sodium content is stated on the label in terms of the number of milligrams (mg) of sodium in the average serving and in each one hundred grams of food.

When dietetic foods are sold across state lines, federal law requires that they have this information. However, when dietetic foods are sold only within a state, they are subject to state laws, which vary widely.

## Booklets on low-sodium diets

The American Heart Association has three booklets with diet and menu information: *Your 500 Milligram Sodium Diet; Your 1000 Milligram Sodium Diet;* and *Your Mild Sodium-Restricted Diet.* All available from American Heart Association, 44 E. 23rd St., New York, N.Y. 10010, but on doctor's request or prescription only.

*Low-Sodium Diets Can Be Delicious* is available from Standard Brands Inc., 625 Madison Ave., New York, N.Y. 10022.

# 11

## Exercise and What
## It Can Do

Most of us don't wear out—we rust out.

We rust out from inactivity and from extra pounds of weight and from the fatty deposits building up inside arteries that clog up the heart and brain. Our power-mechanized lives, with their labor-saving devices, the power steering and power brakes on our automobiles, the push-buttons and switches, and the lure of TV to sit watching sports (rather than performing in them), and very likely munching snacks or drinking, all induce physiological "rust."

There is increasing medical opinion that hearts and other body organs fare better in people who get regular exercise and remain physically fit. Lack of physical activity is regarded as an extra risk adding to the damaging effects of high blood pressure.

The medical profession does not have as much data about the importance of exercise as it does about cigarette smoking or cholesterol. But we do have some data which indicate that regular exercise, of the right kind, is good for you. If you have high blood pressure, a few studies indicate that exercise can often help to lower it. If you have normal pressure, exercise is good as one more means of reducing your risk of death from a heart attack or stroke.

## Can the person with high blood pressure do exercise?

He not only can, but should. However, if there has already been damage to the heart, then a program of activity must be chosen more carefully. Exercise is still good, but it should be gradual and steady. Spurts of strenuous exercise and exertion, such as shoveling snow or singles tennis, can strain the heart and cause a heart attack in the vulnerable person. If you have heart damage, you still need exercise, but you should plan it with the advice of your physician.

## Can regular exercise reduce blood pressure?

Although there is still some controversy about this, a number of studies have shown that regular exercise can bring blood pressure down somewhat, particularly if it has been only mildly high.

A Swedish research team studied a group of men with borderline high blood pressure. Some had been on blood pressure drugs, some had not. They pedaled a stationary bicycle one hour three times a week for several weeks. The director of the project, Dr. R. Sannerstedt of the University Hospital of Göteborg, reported at the International Society on Hypertension that both heart rate and blood pressure were lowered.

Dr. Fred Kasch of San Diego, California, worked with a group of men, aged fifty and over, and after a training program of exercise their blood pressures went down from an average of 155/103 to an average of 144/94.

Dr. Kenneth H. Cooper, author of *Aerobics*, the book

about the U.S. Air Force exercises, says persons who have maintained the aerobics exercise program have had a drop in blood pressure.

Drs. Gaston Choquette and Ronald J. Ferguson, of the University of Montreal, also studied long-term physical conditioning in middle-aged men with borderline hypertension. In 165 men, a six-month physical conditioning program produced drops of blood pressure in both normotensive men and in men with slightly high pressures, but those with high blood pressure had greater drops. The conditioning program consisted of weekly two hour sessions of calisthenics, jogging, volleyball, and swimming. The men were also advised to perform daily calisthenics at home.

Dr. Joseph A. Bonanno and colleagues at the University of California at Davis, studied thirty-nine policemen and firemen. After twelve weeks of training there was "a significant reduction" in blood pressure. Also, Dr. Bonanno said, the exercise training led to a substantial improvement in general physical fitness, with increases in oxygen consumption and increase in work capacity at a lower heart rate.

At San Diego State College Exercise Laboratory, a group of hypertensive men were placed on a program of calisthenics plus half an hour of walking and jogging twice a week. After six months mean blood pressure had dropped from an unhealthy 159/105 to a better 146/93.

At Vanderbilt University School of Medicine, more than one hundred men, aged twenty-five to sixty, were worked out at training sessions of an hour each. Calisthenics, walking, jogging and running. Three quarters stuck through the six months program. Blood pressures fell significantly.

At 5:30 in the morning in Los Angeles, on the shoreline of Palos Verdes Peninsula, you will see a group of physicians gathering who firmly believe in the value of exercise on the heart and blood pressure. They meet regularly, and run about one hundred miles per week. One of the most dedicated of the group is Dr. Thomas Bassler, of South Bay Hospital in Redondo Beach.

In an article about the doctor marathoners in *Medical Tribune* he said he first became interested in exercise and heart disease when working as a pathologist in the Los Angeles County Medical Examiner's office.

"I first began to notice the tiny coronary arteries of polio victims and other invalids during autopsies," he said. "These people were not capable of exercising significantly, and I noticed how especially small [their coronary arteries] appeared when compared to those of people who lived in rural areas where there were few roads and who must, of necessity, exercise a great deal."

Dr. Bassler points out that 50 percent of U.S. physicians die from coronary heart disease, and he and his wife plan to continue running so as not to be one of those statistics.

"One of our marathoning colleagues, Dr. Richard Steiner, has done some studies on our group," he says. "From his observations and those of others, it appears that long-distance running can give you a teen-age cholesterol level, remodel your lungs, lower your blood pressure, and reduce your pulse rate two beats for every thousand miles."

So exercise, performed regularly, can help reduce blood pressure, and we recommend it as one more way to keep pressure down.

Besides, it makes you look better and feel better and it's fun.

### What kinds of exercises are advised?

Plain walking for one, over increasing distances, building up to a brisk pace. And jogging or tennis if you are in good enough shape for them, or develop into it. Dancing is good exercise. So is table tennis. There is a wide choice.

Whatever exercise you choose, it should be within the limits of your capability, now and later. You are not an invalid, sidelined for life. You can exercise wisely, and enjoy it. Talk to your doctor about what you can do safely, how frequently, and how much.

### What about competitive sports, like tennis?

Some doctors advise avoiding competitive sports if you have high blood pressure. Much depends upon your own personality.

But your exercising should be fun. And it should be regular, encouraged from childhood on, continued throughout adult life.

Whether competitive sports will raise your blood pressure depends more on your reactions when you play than what you play. Any exertion with tension can raise the blood pressure. You can play tennis loose and play golf loose or you can do the same sort of thing in a tense, tight, competitive way.

This is one advantage to taking blood pressure at home—you can take a reading after any questionable activity and see if it raised your pressure, and whether your pressure stayed up or went right down again.

### Walking down the avenue

Just plain walking can be a great exercise.

According to a study at the Physical Fitness Research Laboratory of Wake Forest University, walking is as good as any exercise, and better than most to improve your appearance, heart and lungs.

The study involved sixteen healthy but sedentary males between the ages of forty and fifty-six, and showed that: walking gave 28 percent more oxygen to the heart, lowered diastolic blood pressure significantly, and increased pulmonary circulation by 15 percent.

And one advantage over jogging is that walkers suffer none of the muscle strains, joint sprains, foot ailments, or heel injuries that joggers do.

So park your car, and get out your walking shoes.


## *Isometric exercises*

The principle of isometric exercises is to pit one muscle or set of muscles against another in pulling or pushing actions.

There is a great deal of uncertainty about isometric exercises. Some physicians consider them beneficial to persons with high blood pressure. Drs. Broino Kiveloff and Olive Huber, of the New York Infirmary and Hunter College, in New York City, have reported lowering of high blood pressure when patients did isometric exercises for six seconds three times a day. The exercise had no effect on normal blood pressures.

Most doctors have reported that isometrics are harmful. One report from England stated that isometrics raised blood pressure to 300 mm Hg. in a normotensive person. Dr. Joseph Hayes of New York Hospital found that isometric exercises increased blood pressure, but did not provide sufficient stress to produce electrocardiograph abnormalities.

Until more data comes in on isometric exercises, we would advise against them. Vigorous walking, jogging, running, bicycling, and swimming are excellent exercises for the person with high blood pressure. Weight lifting and isometrics are best left alone. Even upper arm exercises like pulling on weights attached to a wall produce large increases in blood pressure and should be avoided.

The exercises thought best for improving circulation are those that involve large muscles actively, such as the leg muscles.

## What about exercise and heart disease?

Studies have also shown that individuals with more physically demanding occupations or leisure time activities generally have a lower incidence of coronary disease than those who are more sedentary, and that cardiovascular function can be dramatically improved by physical training programs for coronary patients.

For example, studies have shown a lower incidence in active bus conductors versus sedentary bus drivers, and in physically active railroad switchmen versus inactive railroad clerks. And a study of ten thousand men in Israel showed men in sedentary occupations were four times more likely to develop heart disease than those who use their muscles to earn their living.

The actual difference in calories spent between the moderately active person and the sedentary person is only in the range of three hundred to five hundred per day. In fact, the very active person seems to be no better off than the moderately active person, when both are compared to the least active person. These findings indicate that activity probably does not have to be excessive to be beneficial.

This was shown nicely in a study just completed by Dr. J. N. Morris of London. He questioned more than sixteen thousand British government workers—who did physically very light work—about their physical activity during leisure hours. When those who developed heart disease were compared with others of like age, diet and other characteristics, it was found that those who did not develop heart disease on the average were more active in leisure hours than those who did develop heart disease. Physical activity —whether it was swimming, walking, or digging in the garden—had a protective effect against heart disease. And it appeared that the length of time spent in the exercising was unrelated to the benefits.

Dr. D. F. Muckle, medical advisor of the Oxford United

Football Club, says that as little as seventeen to twenty minutes a day of exercise for three days a week can make the difference.

"Exercise tones the muscles, stimulates the circulation, and helps to avoid overweight," the American Heart Association says. "It tends to reduce the risk of heart disease, because arteries which supply blood to the heart improve their efficiency when exercise makes demands on them."

"The average American settles down at about age twenty-five to a life of physical inactivity," says the AHA. "When he does get exercise, he tends to overdo it—and strains his out-of-shape body."

The association recommends a brisk walk of about two miles every day as an ideal program, plus sports such as swimming, bicycling, skiing, skating, golf, tennis, bowling, and dancing. Whatever the program, they say, it should begin slowly, build up gradually, and continue daily if possible.

### *Exercise for the person who has severe heart disease or has had a heart attack*

Even the person who has had a heart attack need not be put on the sidelines of non-exercise. In fact, many physicians are setting up regular exercise programs for their heart patients to follow to build up the strength of their hearts again.

In Cleveland, Dr. Herman Hellerstein has worked with 260 heart disease patients, some of whom had heart attacks and some of whom had chest pains, but not actual heart attacks. After a physical fitness program, the patients were able to perform muscular effort more efficiently with lower heart rate, lower blood pressure, and greater oxygen capacity, Dr. Hellerstein reported. Physical fitness was significantly improved and sustained during the three-year program in 64 percent of the patients with heart disease, and the death rate was lower.

At the Mayo Clinic, Dr. Charles Kennedy reported results from a one-year exercise program for men with severe coronary artery disease. At the beginning of the program, he said, all patients had angina. At the end of the year, the angina was either considerably reduced or completely gone. The exercises consisted of calisthenics, walking, jogging, volleyball, and swimming.

In Vermont, he said, the Preventive Heart Reconditioning Foundation is setting up a center just for rehabilitation of heart attack patients to prevent the recurrence of attacks. The course will include exercise programs and advice on following a low-fat, low-calorie diet, giving up smoking, and counteracting stress and tension.

### *Who should follow a restricted exercise program?*

For anyone who hasn't exercised for a long time, a physical checkup is in order before he or she becomes a casualty of weekend athletics. The most common test is to have the person run on a treadmill, then to check his heart with an electrocardiogram for any irregularities. A general physical examination also will be given, and a chest x-ray may be taken. The car may look good on the outside, but we want to make sure it's in good condition inside, too.

If a person has congestive heart failure, upsets in rhythm of the heart, or other evidence of heart disease, he needs to go easier with exercise. As a matter of fact, if you have heart enlargement or heart disease of any kind, your exercise program must be individualized. Have your doctor plan your exercise program in every detail. Ask him specifically whether you can do housework, can mow the lawn, walk to the bus, play golf, or work in your garden; ask what exercise or activities you can't do, and be sure you understand his answers.

What's more, it is particularly important if you have heart disease to have a warm-up and cool-off period each time you exercise, and your activity should be increased in a slower, more carefully supervised manner than the person who has no heart problems. There should be a very gradual increase in activity, with no sudden exertions—like four hours of tennis singles or snow shoveling on weekends after a week of sitting at the desk.

### Exercise and losing weight

One of the bonuses of exercise is that it burns up calories. It not only firms you up, but it helps you get rid of excess weight. Weight loss is good for high blood pressure and is good for increasing your odds of avoiding a heart attack.

Anything that takes calories out of your body's calorie bank helps. One pound of fat represents thirty-five hundred stored-up or "banked" calories.

A brisk walk will use up about three hundred calories in an hour, so walking just an extra fifteen minutes a day can make you lose one pound in forty-seven days, or about eight pounds in a year. Playing a half hour of handball over twelve days burns up a pound. A half hour everyday all year and you've lost more than 30 pounds.

Extra weight is most likely to accumulate steadily, bit by bit, through too much food and too little exercise. Bit by bit, but steadily, can be the best way to take it off, too.

Of course the very best exercise of all is to firmly push yourself away from the table before you take a second helping.

Many people don't realize that as we grow older, our body metabolism slows down. If, for example, a twenty-year-old, 135-pound man eats and exercises exactly the same amount until he is fifty-five, he will weigh fifty pounds more just because his metabolism has slowed down.

## Calorie expenditures

Weight gain and weight loss depend not only upon caloric intake but also upon calories used. The body uses calories simply to maintain its functioning. Beyond that, energy needs—caloric expenditures—depend upon the kind of work and leisure time activities that a person engages in.

For convenience, various activities have been grouped into five general types in the following table.*

| Calories expended per hour | *Type of activity* |
|---|---|
| 80–100 | *Sedentary*: Includes such activities as reading, writing, watching TV or movies, sewing, playing cards, typing, general office work, other activities carried out while sitting that involve little or no movement of the arms. |
| 110–160 | *Light*: Includes food preparation and cooking, dishwashing, dusting, washing small garments, ironing, personal care, slow walking, office work and activities done while standing and requiring some movement of the arms, and rapid typing, collating, etc., done while sitting. |
| 170–240 | *Moderate*: Includes bedmaking, mopping, scrubbing, sweeping, polishing and waxing, light gardening, carpentry, moderately fast walking, other activities carried out while standing and calling for moderate arm movements, and any activity done while seated that involves fairly vigorous arm motions. |

* Courtesy United States Department of Agriculture (*Food and Your Weight*)

250–350  *Vigorous*: Includes heavy scrubbing and wax-
ing, hanging out clothes, stripping beds, other
heavy work, fast walking, gardening.

350–up  *Strenuous*: Includes swimming, tennis, running,
bicycling, dancing, skiing, football. Actually,
depending upon speed, running may call for
calorie expenditures of from 800 to 1,300 an
hour; swimming, 300 to 1,000; rowing, 1,000
to 1,500; cycling, 150–600. A very fast walk
(5.3 miles an hour) may consume as many as
565 calories an hour.

# 12

# *Kicking the Cigarette Habit*

As we were sitting in the meeting of the Advisory Committee of the High Blood Pressure Education Program in Washington, we suddenly realized that not one person in the room—and there must have been fifty people there—was smoking.

Later, whether over cocktails, doing tapings, conducting interviews, it was the same thing—none of the men and women we encountered who were involved in treatment of high blood pressure or heart disease was ever seen smoking.

We asked them about it. Said one doctor: "As soon as I read the Surgeon General's report on the effect of smoking on cancer and heart disease, I stopped smoking." Another, who used to be a real chainsmoker ("I smoked in the shower."), said he stopped when a checkup showed he had blood pressure twenty points higher than it should have been. Another said, "The first day I coughed up blood was the last day I smoked a cigarette. That was ten years ago, and I haven't smoked since."

We can look at statistics like those in a previous chapter on how smoking increases your risk of disease. If you have high blood pressure and smoke, your chances of having a heart attack are five times higher than otherwise. Your chances of having a stroke sixteen times higher. But what really convinces us is when we see all those doctors who know about high blood pressure and heart disease, and they don't smoke!

What do doctors tell their patients who have high blood pressure?

"Cigarette smoking should be prohibited," says Dr. Ray W. Gifford, head of the department of hypertension at Cleveland Clinic Foundation in Ohio. Writing in *The Hypertension Handbook*, a book on high blood pressure for physicians prepared by Merck Sharp and Dohme, the pharmaceutical company, Dr. Gifford says, "It makes little sense to treat one risk factor for coronary disease (hypertension) and ignore others (i.e., cigarette smoking) which are almost equally important." But he says he permits cigar and pipe smoking, "provided that the patient does not inhale."

We agree.

### What should I do about smoking?

If you have high blood pressure, give up smoking. Don't just cut down; stop completely. Giving up cigarettes is one of the most positive life-saving things you can do at any time. And that's particularly true when you have high blood pressure.

And, of course, there will be the added benefits of less risk of getting any of the many other diseases associated with smoking, including lung cancer.

### How hard is it really to give up smoking?

Some people find it a terrible ordeal, a bitter battle that takes every ounce of their willpower. Others find that once they really make up their minds to quit, the battle isn't really all that difficult. And that's the secret—to *really* make up your mind to do it.

There are now some 30 million ex-cigarette smokers in the United States. Nearly two-thirds of adult men and women in the United States do not smoke.

### Do filters make cigarettes safe?

The American Heart Association says, "Most filters now in use reduce only moderately the amount of harmful substances in cigarette smoke." And they say there is no such thing as a cigarette which has been proved "safe."

### Is there any risk in smoking cigarettes if you don't inhale?

It is true that the smoker who doesn't inhale has lower risks than the inhaler, but very few steady smokers do not inhale. Often, a smoker can inhale without being aware of it. Even the noninhaler absorbs some of the nicotine in cigarettes and retains some of the tars in his mouth.

### What about withdrawal symptoms and side effects?

There may be some temporary side effects as you stop smoking. You may have constipation for a while, or urinate frequently, or you may become shaky, tense, irritable, or depressed. You may start to gain weight. Some people find that their coughing actually increases for the first week.

Some of the symptoms are withdrawal symptoms. Other symptoms appear to be the result of anxiety and tension. If you have psychological distress, you will find the first forty-eight hours are the critical period. If you have shortness of breath, tightness in the chest, visual disturbances, sweating, headaches, gastrointestinal complaints, don't let them alarm you. It is simply that your body is actively readjusting to the non-smoking state. These symptoms will all pass in a week or two, and are worth sweating through for the overall benefits. Just keep reminding yourself of all the good effects that stopping smoking is having on you.

Helen M. stopped and found her cough disappeared, her sense of taste and smell improved, her skin circulation improved, with her complexion looking better almost immediately. And she was less tired and more alert.

You usually have an increase in sexual energy, too. You will have more wind for running, tennis, or other exercise. Patients with chronic bronchitis, emphysema, or asthma improve almost overnight and are able to breath much more easily.

And most important to you, your non-smoking will have improved the health of your heart and blood vessels.

### *If you have smoked for years, does quitting now really help?*

Yes, even if you have smoked for ten or twenty years. If you quit now, it will almost immediately help your heart and blood vessels. Studies show that even after only one year of non-smoking, the chances of having a heart attack or stroke drop significantly.

The longer you stay off the cigarettes, of course, the more beneficial the results.

### *Can you give me a plan to follow for breaking the cigarette habit?*

Dr. Donald T. Fredrickson, a leader in establishing smoking withdrawal clinics, has this to say: "Every smoker can conquer the cigarette habit irrespective of how addicted, how defeated or discouraged he may feel or how many times he has temporarily stopped only to fall off the wagon. This is true because cigarette smoking is a *habit*. A habit is learned behavior. Learning to be a smoker is like learning anything else. If one can learn to be a smoker, one can learn not to smoke. To conquer the cigarette habit once and for all one must learn in reverse. To succeed one trains himself in nonsmoking the same way that he was trained in smoking.

"Success with any program of training requires a willingness and determination to carry through. One's reasons for wanting to stop must be strong and important."

In giving up cigarettes, says Fredrickson, one should adopt an attitude that is positive and self-reinforcing. "Stopping smoking is not a minus, a taking away, rather it is a plus—building into one's personality a new exciting dimension of self-control."

### Where do I start?

The first thing you need to do is decide which method of giving up cigarettes best fits you and your personality.

Floyd T. has pride in his strong willpower and enjoys challenging himself to a battle. Giving up cigarettes successfully proved to him that he had self-control, that he was completely in command and master of his own destiny and habits.

Other people find willpower is not the answer. For them the answer to breaking the old habit is a learning of new habits, new patterns. They need to be relaxed, and then with patience and perseverance they talk to themselves, to slowly change their feelings about cigarettes, and then with self-suggestion gradually change their habits also. Just as they taught themselves to smoke, they now teach themselves *not* to smoke.

Think about what would be best for you: The cold turkey method of immediate and total quitting based on willpower, or working slowly with self-suggestion. They are equally good methods. It's simply a matter of choosing which one is best for you.

Whichever method you choose, it is important that you think of becoming a non-smoker as a good thing, that you think of it not as a self-denial, not as something to feel sorry for yourself about, but as something positive, and constructive, with great rewards.

### Helpful hints for kicking the habit

Once you've decided whether cold turkey or slow-and-gradual is the best method for you, then move ahead immediately.

To help you form your new habit of not smoking, here are hints that have been collected from doctors, psychologists, directors of smoking withdrawal clinics, and from former smokers themselves. Read through the list and decide right now the items that you think will be most helpful to you. Then do them.

• Throw away your cigarettes immediately, and give away your lighter. Put away the ashtrays.

• Use substitutes. Drink frequent glasses of water and juices. Nibble fruit, celery, carrots, cookies, candy, clove, bits of ginger. Chew gum.

• Brush your teeth, use mouthwashes and cough drops frequently until you get over the first few weeks.

• Double the number of cigarettes you smoke the day before you quit. Your body will revolt at the increase so much that quitting will be a relief.

• Don't carry change so you can't use cigarette machines.

• Each day, put aside the money you have been spending on cigarettes. Watch it add up at fifty cents to a dollar a day. That reminds you of the waste, and gives you money for something else you want.

• Think of the money you have spent smoking in past years. If you've smoked two packs a day for 21 years, for example, that's 300,000 cigarettes. All in a row, they'd stretch 17 miles. At five minutes per cigarette, you used up one thousand days smoking them. Buying them cost you over five thousand dollars.

• Remind yourself each day why you HATE cigarettes. Think of the shocking risk of disease, decrease in the taste of food, bad breath, morning-after ashtrays, effects on children, the fact that you may—if you continue smoking—lose many years of life. Make a list and look at it whenever you feel you need a cigarette.

• Chart your smoking habits, making a daily record of how many cigarettes you smoke so you can see how much progress you make as you eliminate the ones you need the least.

• Switch from the cigarettes you like to ones that you do not like.

• Before you light up, ask yourself, "Do I really want this cigarette or am I just acting out of habit?" You may be amazed at how many cigarettes you don't really want.

• Make it a real effort to get at your cigarettes. Wrap them in several sheets of paper, or place them in a tightly covered box. Buy only one pack of cigarettes at a time, never a carton. Carry your cigarettes in a different place. At work, give them to your secretary or put them in another room.

• If you're right-handed, try smoking with your left hand to make it more awkward.

• Break up the habit patterns that you associate with smoking. Avoid people and things that you usually connect with smoking. For the first difficult days spend as much time as possible in libraries or other places where smoking is forbidden. Go to the no-smoking section at movies and on the train. When possible, stay away from friends who are heavy smokers for the first two weeks.

• It sometimes helps to set quitting day as the first day of a new routine or new environment—the first day on a new job, at a new house, on a date with a new person. Or give up smoking while on vacation when daily habits are not a factor.

• When you need a cigarette, keep an unlighted one in your mouth. Or handle a cigarette, but don't light it.

• When you feel like you must have a smoke, take a shower. It's hard to smoke in the shower, even though some die-hards (you will excuse the expression) do it.

• Get plenty of sleep during the first few weeks so that you will cut down on nervousness or irritability.

• Use your lungs. Deep breathing exercises whenever you feel the need for a cigarette can be very calming. Sometimes the craving will go away in just three or four minutes.

• If you usually have a cigarette with a drink or with a cup of coffee, then eliminate coffee and alcohol for the first few weeks. Drink fruit juices, milk, lots of water.

• If you are largely a social smoker and feel that smoking makes you feel closer to others, more welcome at a party, go to a party and don't smoke. You'll find that people like and respect you for more important reasons than whether you smoke a cigarette.

• Strenuous physical activity can be very helpful, particularly in working off the irritation or tension from not having a cigarette in the mouth. Stretching exercises, calisthenics, or long walks can also be relaxing.

• Inhalers—ones that clear sinuses—may help tide you over the first few days.

• If you have a specific pattern that you follow after dinner, change it. Read a book instead of a newspaper. Sit in a different chair, do some household task you have been putting off, take your dog or child out for a walk.

• Reward yourself: Be sure that you have your favorite

food on quitting day. Give yourself all the things that you like best—except cigarettes.

## *If you want to do it gradually*

If you are going to cut down gradually, then set a schedule to reduce a specific number of cigarettes you smoke each day or week, or just smoke half of each cigarette. Or don't smoke during certain hours.

Or stop for just one day at a time. Promise yourself twenty-four hours of freedom from cigarettes, and when the day is over, make a commitment for one more day. And another. And another.

With any of these methods, the idea is gradually to cut down more and more and then to set a final target date after which you will *absolutely* not have any more!

## *Other sources of help*

If you feel that you need further help, you might consider getting some support through group sessions, smoking withdrawal clinics, or hypnosis.

To find out if there are any smoking clinics in your area—many are free—check with your local chapter of the American Heart Association, American Cancer Society, or American Lung Association. There are also groups who charge, such as Smoke Watchers and Smoke Enders, and the Seventh Day Adventists. The American Health Foundation has a program in New York, as does Human Research Laboratories.

*Helping People to Stop Smoking Cigarettes*, a kit for groups wishing to establish programs, is available, free, from the American Cancer Society. Consult your telephone book for the office nearest you, or write to the ACS at P.O. Box 218, Fairview, N.J. 07022.

The *Smoker's Self-Testing Kit* (HEW publication No. 72-7506) is available for ten cents from the Superintendent of Documents, U.S. Government Printing Office, Washington, D.C. 20402.

*What Everyone Should Know About Smoking and Heart Disease* is available from the American Heart Association, 44 E. 23rd Street, New York, N.Y. 10010.

### What about anti-smoking drugs?

The stop-smoking preparations that are available fall into two categories: nicotine substitutes which are primarily lobeline compounds, and spicy lozenges which give you a taste in your mouth which is supposed to be offensive when you smoke. It is not known whether they really have a physical effect or whether the effects are primarily psychological.

### Can hypnosis help?

Preliminary reports from several investigators are encouraging. However, if you decide to try hypnosis as an aid, be sure to be hypnotized only by a qualified and responsible professional.

### How long will the craving to smoke last?

The craving to smoke is temporary. Usually within days the acute craving begins to subside, and after two or three weeks there is only an occasional desire to light up.

### *What can I do to avoid gaining weight when I stop smoking?*

Many who stop smoking do not gain weight. Some even lose weight during withdrawal.

Usually if weight gain occurs, it is minimal, and most ex-smokers find that once the acute urge to smoke subsides they are able to bring their weight back to normal with little difficulty.

# 13

# The Role of Stress and What You Can Do About It

One of the leading cardiologists in the field of high blood pressure told us a story about his mother. When he moved to a distant city, she developed really high blood pressure, up to 240 systolic, very dangerous. The doctor caring for her was worried. He tried every drug in the book, but nothing seemed to keep her pressure down. When the son started calling his mother every evening on the telephone, her pressure almost immediately went down to normal and stayed there.

While this is a case history of only one person, there are many other similar stories. Anxiety and stress do appear to be related to high blood pressure. But the question is how much and in exactly what way? How important is stress compared to other factors? We all have anxieties and stresses. What makes one person get high blood pressure and not another?

Surprise, fear, and sexual excitement may make your blood pressure go up. And it can zoom up ten to twenty points in just a matter of seconds when you become excited or angry or frightened. But it usually comes right down again once the episode is over. And the temporary rise doesn't appear to do any harm.

But apparently in some people pressure may stay up after the stress is over or if they remain under persistent or continuing stress. Day after day, continuing problems at work and at home, debts or other worries may provoke a slow, steady rise in pressure. And some studies indicate that the feeling of being trapped in life, frustrated by seemingly unsolvable situations, can be a powerful force in boosting blood pressure. For example, the prevalence of high blood pressure is higher in blacks than whites. Is this due to physical reasons or is it due to the constant frustration and stress of black life?

In addition, in some people who already have high blood pressure, severe anxiety can make it worse. But the anxiety doesn't *cause* the high pressure in these people, it only aggravates it further.

The current belief among many researchers now is that some people have a predisposition to hypertension in the way their body reacts to stress. Emotional stress triggers their high blood pressure just as other factors can trigger the high pressure in other people. And although emotional stress may be important, the calm, cool, collected person can be dying of hypertension just as easily as the excitable one. Both relaxed and tense persons can be subject to the disease.

### *Just what physical effect does stress produce?*

Stress will increase outpouring of certain hormones which, like adrenalin and other chemicals, act on the nervous system, heart, blood vessels, and various organs. Blood vessels, for example, react to stress by contracting, becoming narrower. This calls for higher pressure to force the blood along.

Different people react differently to stress. One may get

intestinal upsets or headaches. Another may develop sweating or palpitations of the heart. Another may have a rise in blood pressure.

And what is stress for one person may not be stress for another. An airplane pilot would find it stressful if called upon to take out someone's appendix. A surgeon's blood pressure might zoom if he had to take control of a jet airplane.

### Can you spot people whose reactions are boosting their blood pressure, even if only temporarily?

No. The overweight, red-faced person may have high pressure, or quite normal pressure. The thin, calm-looking individual may have high pressure, but appear quite normal.

The busy tycoon, pounding his fist on his desk, is not necessarily driving his blood pressure up. The man in trouble may be the one who bottles up his emotions.

### What stress can do to you—the research

How much can the pressures and tensions of life affect our blood pressure?

At Munich University in Germany, two tiny tree shrews are caged together. They are two adult males, one stronger than the other. They fight and are separated. The beaten one crouches in a neighboring cage, hairs up, eyes constantly watching the victor. Every few days they are put together again. The loser, within a few days, dies not from wounds, but from kidney failure. The kidney damage in the defeated shrews, says researcher Professor Dietrich von Holst, is just like the kidney damage in patients who die from malignant hypertension.

At the University of Southern California School of

Medicine, Dr. James P. Henry and his colleagues take mice as soon as they are weaned and put them into isolation jars away from others. At the age of four months they are returned to the rest of the group with other mice that have been isolated. Subsequent socializing is a failure and high blood pressure develops almost immediately. Other studies have shown that rats and mice have sustained elevated pressure when exposed to stresses such as noise and flashing lights.

Does stress affect blood pressure in man as well?

There is some evidence that it does. One classic study involves men who were asked to work arithmetic problems in their heads while they were harassed by a constantly ticking metronome. Their heart rate and blood pressure both went up. Blood pressure has also been shown to go up in subjects during stressful interviews, and at times of anger provoked in a laboratory.

Epidemics of high blood pressure during stress occurs among soldiers during battle. Over 30 percent of one group had blood pressures of 180 millimeters or more. It took about two months for it to return to normal.

When people with high blood pressure and people with normal blood pressure are exposed to the same amount of stress under controlled laboratory conditions, those with high blood pressure will have much greater rises in pressure.

One study was done of several dozen men who were in danger of losing their jobs at a large company. The men's pressure remained elevated during the entire time they were worried about their jobs, when they lost them, when they were out of work, and during the beginning of new jobs. Once accustomed to the jobs and secure again, their blood pressures dropped back to normal.

It has been shown in a number of studies that under emotional stress, pressures can rise anywhere from fifty to more than eighty points, and a number of case histories have been reported, similar to that of the cardiologist's mother, whose high blood pressure dropped once stress was removed. Another such case was an unhappily married woman who spent her years in frustration, without love or satisfaction. Her blood pressure was dangerously high until she obtained a divorce, found a man she really cared for, and remarried. Then her blood pressure returned to normal. High blood pressure is often seen during divorce proceedings or when a family member dies.

### Moment-to-moment measurements

In the past, one of the problems in trying to investigate the role of stress was that there was no way to measure what was happening to the blood pressure on an instantaneous basis as events actually took place in a subject's life. Now a portable blood pressure measuring apparatus has been devised to do that and is showing that stress does play a role, at least in temporary pressure rises. This kind of equipment has shown, for example, that a pilot who had to wait four hours for mechanical troubles to his plane to be fixed had a great increase in pressure, which promptly dropped when he could get on with his job. Another pilot showed a huge rise in pressure when he overheard someone make a disparaging remark about him.

Apparently, says Dr. Maurice Sokolow, it is not the nature of the event itself that is of critical importance, "but rather the individual's perception of the event and, accordingly, his emotional responses to it."

At the University of California Medical School in San Francisco, Dr. Sokolow has studied more than one hundred men and women with portable recorders. Measurements indicate that the more contentment the person reports during the time of blood pressure recordings, the lower the blood pressure and pulse rate. During times of anxiety, or when pressed by time, pressures were higher.

"The more severe the hypertension, the more likely the patient is to report anxiety, depression, or hostility," Dr.

Sokolow says. But he adds, "Is the patient hypertensive because he is anxious, or anxious because he is hypertensive?"

The portable recorders are also useful in helping the doctor and patient pinpoint those situations that are particularly stressful and which the patient should avoid.

"We had one businessman," Dr. Sokolow says, "whose blood pressure went up whenever he was on the phone trying to persuade someone to do something. When he was interacting personally with someone, his pressure was not as high. Other people, who might love to talk on the phone but can't deal with people face to face, might react the other way around."

### *Is there a typical high blood pressure type of personality?*

Generally speaking, no. It is a popular misconception that a hypertensive patient is a nervous, compulsive, never-resting perfectionist who cannot sit still. This is not necessarily the case.

Some people with high blood pressure may be this type, whereas others are relaxed, well-adjusted, quiet, and calm.

Psychological factors and types of behavior do seem to play a role in some people, but not all.

Suppression of emotions as a possible factor was studied at Michael Reese Hospital in Chicago. There, persons with normal blood pressure were exposed to anger-provoking situations. Those who bottled up their anger had large increases in pressure, those who expressed their anger had much less increase.

Some people seem to react to even mild life stresses with an excessive rise in blood pressure. They are called hyper-reactors. Their bodies, somehow, seem to respond to daily life as if it were a series of emergencies. Evidence indicates that they tend in time to develop full-blown high blood pressure.

## *Personality and heart attacks*

A person's reactions to the problems of life do seem to be a factor in who is most likely to get heart attacks and strokes.

Research by Drs. Meyer Friedman and Ralph Roseman indicates that persons with a high-pressured, aggressive personality have a higher risk of developing coronary heart disease. The aggressive, hard-driving individual—what physicians call the Type A personality—was found more often in a group of men who had heart disease than the person who is easygoing and not always racing to meet a deadline.

The coronary-prone individual, says the American Heart Association, "often demonstrates an excessive drive, a sense of time urgency, and an immoderate emotional attitude or reaction to stress. Instead of calmly solving his problems by discussing them with someone, or trying a new approach, he overreacts to these problems, becoming mentally and physically immobile and perhaps even incapable of resolving them. He is like a machine running with its brakes on and with the pressure unable to escape from the engine."

Scientists have tried to make up a questionnaire that will detect Type A personalities and other psychological characteristics that might be predictive of future heart attacks. When men and women were scored on a 155-item psychological questionnaire, there did seem to be certain responses that stood out as being predictive of heart attacks. For example, people who said they were often completely worn out and felt they were in poor health most of the time were twice as likely later to get heart attacks as those who answered "no" to these questions. But other responses showed little or no relationship. For example, none of the responses to questions dealing with worry and tension were statistically significant. Some were actually in direct opposition to the predicted direction.

Discussing the questions, Dr. Gary Friedman, who gave the test to several hundred patients in Oakland, California, said: "Some of the responses would appear to contradict the popular notion that worry and tension lead to heart attacks."

"We could not confirm the Type A hypothesis in our data and we had to conclude that if our questionnaire was predictive it was not because it was measuring Type A personality," he said. However, he added that this did not disprove the Type A idea because the trait is better measured by observing a person's behavior rather than having him answer questions.

The two most predictive responses—feeling worn out and feeling in poor health most of the time—are generally thought by psychologists to be evidence of emotional drain, indicating a person is in a state of physical and mental exhaustion due to serious long-term emotional conflicts. But it occurred to the psychologists that "some of these patients who were destined to develop myocardial infarctions already had some coronary disease symptoms, and that what they were telling us is that they were physically ill . . . in other words, when a person says that he has been tired and worn out or that he often has spells of trembling or shaking he may be indicating that he is already sick with atherosclerosis."

So, results are confusing.

One other fascinating study is going on at the Washington University Medical Center in St. Louis. There, preliminary studies indicate that blood pressure and heart attacks follow definite biological rhythms. And heart attacks seem to occur at the times when a person's regular rhythms are at their lowest points. Some investigators are suggesting that by charting out these rhythms and avoiding strain and dangerous activity during these low periods, heart attacks might often be averted.

## Why now?

Why does a person have a heart attack on a certain day? Why not the month before or a year later?

Often, says Dr. Abraham Lenzner, of Cornell University Medical College, the patient has been enmeshed in family, economic, or other problems, in the face of which he feels helpless and hopeless.

He and a Cornell cardiologist, Dr. Alfred L. Aronson, now at Yale, worked together for five years interviewing more than one hundred heart attack patients within the first few days of their attacks.

Most patients revealed that the onset of their coronary episode was related to mixtures of emotional, psychological, social, and economic problems. One man, for example, said his marriage was intolerable. His five-year-old son was the only person who mattered to him. If he committed suicide, he would leave nothing. However, if he smoked himself to death, his insurance would safely pass to his son.

Dr. Bernard Lown, with a team of psychologists and cardiologists at Harvard, is also exploring how stresses may provoke a special kind of heart attack, where sudden death occurs from upsets in heart rhythm. The team, working with dogs, is finding that stresses can greatly increase the effect of small upsets in rhythm that ordinarily would cause no problem. Dr. Lown has just returned from Moscow, where he has reached preliminary agreement with Russians to coordinate studies on sudden death in both countries.

## Linking life's stresses to illness

Changes that happen to you in life, good and bad, seem to affect whether and when you develop many illnesses. Drs.

Thomas Holmes and Minoru Masuda, psychiatrists at the University of Washington in Seattle, have devised a scale to help predict stress-related illness. They find that death of a spouse or other family member, divorce, separation, and a jail term were all high on the scale for most people in producing stress, although such events as marriage, pregnancy, job change, moving, buying a house, or getting an award could also produce stress.

Whether good or bad, life changes appear "to have relevance to the causation of disease, time of onset of disease, and severity of disease," Dr. Holmes says.

Point values were given to such events. In eighty-eight patients studied, 93 percent of all major illnesses were associated with a clustering of life changes whose values totalled at least 150 points in a year, Dr. Holmes reported.

But a cluster of changes or a major crisis did not *always* produce illness. Of persons with life changes totalling 150 to 199 points, 37 percent had an illness. When changes totalled 200 to 299, 51 percent had illness. When changes totalled over 300, 79 percent became ill.

These are the life events that appeared to affect health, with the point values the scientists assigned for them.

| LIFE EVENT | VALUE |
|---|---|
| Death of spouse | 100 |
| Divorce | 73 |
| Marital separation | 65 |
| Jail term | 63 |
| Death of close family member | 63 |
| Personal injury or illness | 53 |
| Marriage | 50 |
| Fired at work | 47 |
| Marital reconciliation | 45 |
| Retirement | 45 |
| Change in health of family member | 44 |

| | |
|---|---|
| Pregnancy | 40 |
| Sex difficulties | 39 |
| Gain of new family member | 39 |
| Business readjustment | 39 |
| Change in financial state | 38 |
| Death of close friend | 37 |
| Change to different line of work | 36 |
| Change in number of arguments with spouse | 35 |
| Mortgage over $10,000 | 31 |
| Foreclosure of mortgage or loan | 30 |
| Change in responsibilities at work | 29 |
| Son or daughter leaving home | 29 |
| Trouble with in-laws | 29 |
| Outstanding personal achievement | 28 |
| Wife begins or stops work | 26 |
| Begin or end school | 26 |
| Change in living conditions | 25 |
| Revision of personal habits | 24 |
| Trouble with boss | 23 |
| Change in work hours or conditions | 20 |
| Change in residence | 20 |
| Change in schools | 20 |
| Change in recreation | 19 |
| Change in church activities | 19 |
| Change in social activities | 18 |
| Mortgage or loan less than $10,000 | 17 |
| Change in sleeping habits | 16 |
| Change in number of family get-togethers | 15 |
| Change in eating habits | 15 |
| Vacation | 13 |
| Christmas | 12 |
| Minor violations of the law | 11 |

### Stress and your job

How much effect does occupational stress have on high blood pressure and other circulatory diseases?

The most classic study is one done on four thousand airport traffic controllers. Their job of guiding hundreds of planes safely in and out of busy airports was shown to bring on high blood pressure and ulcers, according to a study in the *Journal of the American Medical Association* by Dr. Sidney Cobb, of the University of Michigan, and Dr. Robert M. Rose, of Boston University Medical School.

The air traffic controllers were found to be four times more likely to develop high blood pressure than second-class airmen whose work involves less stress.

Also the frequency of high blood pressure was found to be in proportion to the volume of traffic at the airport. Those in the sometimes frantically busy big city airports had more high blood pressure, while the tower men in smaller airports with relatively few landings and takeoffs had less high blood pressure.

Blood pressures and cholesterol levels go up in medical students at exam time, and in tax accountants as April 15th approaches.

Another study at the University of Michigan, done by psychologists Louise S. Hauenstein and Ernest Harburg, showed that unhappiness with housework was positively related to blood pressure for housewives, and was especially related to tension about housework and low self-ratings of accomplishment in running the house.

Also, at Duke University, psychologist James S. House found that workers who have a low degree of occupational self-esteem and who were not satisfied with their jobs had more heart disease than others.

## Twentieth-century tensions

Cavemen had stresses—saber-toothed tigers, bears, and cold, hungry winters. Roman soldiers and builders of the pyramids had problems, and so did pioneers settling the West. What makes our current society so different that high blood pressure and heart attacks and strokes have become epidemics raging through our population?

Is it hostility felt at home, at work, or on the street? Is it the mechanization and depersonalization of our world? Is it the very lack of activity that machines have brought on with their mass-manufactured comforts and conveniences? Is it a sense of frustration and helplessness that in our complex society we no longer have any control over what happens to our country, to the future of mankind, or even to our own family?

Is it that we have lost the supports that helped people in earlier times—religious faith, frameworks of tradition, closeness of family and community, a sense of place in a social order? Is it the loss of sense of worth in work, in pride of craftsmanship and contribution to the world in doing a job? Is it the constant moving about in jobs that makes us lose our sense of belonging? Is it the endless competition for status and success? Is it the loss of meaning in our personal lives, the lack of close communication with someone we love?

Perhaps it can be any one of them, or all of them.

One theory is that any of these things can set our adrenalin going, pouring hormones into our bloodstream, constricting our blood vessels, mobilizing our muscles for action. We are ready for battle, but all we ever seem to go to battle with is paper clips.

Some researchers believe people are more prone to hypertension when they have no control over the stresses imposed on them. If they have some control over what is happening to them, the tendency to high pressure is decreased.

Dr. George DeLeon has shown that not only will blood pressure go up when a light goes on and a shock is given, but it will also go up from anxiety and anticipation just from the light going on—with no shock. In fact, anxiety alone produced high blood pressure for a longer time than the electric shock itself did.

Dr. Charles Curry, of Howard University in Washington, D.C., believes stress is one of the reasons for the higher blood pressure in blacks. He does not discount heredity or heavy salt in the diet but feels high stress in our discriminatory society is an added factor in blacks.

"Black people are confronted with many stress situations that would be expected to elevate the blood pressure," he says. "I am anxiously awaiting an instrument with which we can monitor blood pressure twenty-four hours a day, because I would like to see what happens to the blood pressure of a black man who cannot get a cab in Chicago because he is black or is not waited on in a restaurant or department store."

Dr. James T. Montgomery, a specialist in internal medicine in Birmingham, Alabama, agrees. "Those of us who are black cannot prove it," he says, "yet we believe that the inward stresses we have suffered from generation to generation have become expressed as hypertension."

### Anxiety hypertension

When severe anxiety over some stress or problem causes high blood pressure, doctors call it, logically enough, "anxiety hypertension." It is often superimposed on top of other high blood pressure, making the pressure even higher, and making management more complicated. In fact, such over-anxiety can also cause your heart to beat faster or upset the rhythm of your heartbeat, causing skipped or extra beats or other irregularity in the beat.

The telltale signs of anxiety are sighing respiration and cold, clammy hands. Unfortunately in some patients, simply knowing they have high blood pressure puts them into such an anxious state, makes them worry so much, that it increases the blood pressure even further. You should be aware that you have high blood pressure—aware enough to take your pills and follow your doctor's advice—but you should not dwell on it or worry about it. This can do no good and can make your blood pressure higher.

### *Does it help to take tranquilizers for anxiety hypertension?*

Yes. But tranquilizers are not effective against other types of hypertension. You need regular high blood pressure medicines for this. Tranquilizers help anxiety hypertension or they may be effective if a person has severe anxiety. Naturally they should only be taken on a doctor's prescription. And, like any drug, only when you really need them.

You should not take tranquilizers if you have liver or kidney damage.

You should not combine tranquilizers with alcohol or with certain cheeses or other drugs such as sleeping pills. The chemical reaction can cause severe depression of the central nervous system. The results can be deadly, literally. It's quite possible for a person to take a tranquilizer, have a few drinks, go home to bed, and be found dead in the morning.

Also, you should not take tranquilizers if you are pregnant or are nursing a newborn baby. The chemicals can go from mother to infant and cause serious trouble. No pregnant woman, as a matter of fact, should ever take any medicine unless she absolutely has to because of the danger of causing birth defects in the developing embryo.

And because they slow down your reactions and often make you drowsy, you should not drive while taking tranquilizers or operate dangerous machinery.

## *Psychotherapy*

If you are deeply disturbed, are anxious and tense, and think it is possible that it is having some effect on your blood pressure, talk it over with your doctor. After you have worked with the other treatments he has advised for you, if you both think that you have undue anxiety that is complicating your high blood pressure, then you might want to consider psychotherapy or group therapy sessions to help you with your anxieties. If you do decide to try this approach, do not depend on it alone to lower your blood pressure. It is only a way to combat excessive anxieties or fears. You must still continue your medical treatment.

## *Are you over-tense?*

Some tensions are natural. They are natural ways of dealing with problems. When there is danger, your adrenalin surges out to meet it.

It is the unneeded tension, the excess tension over unimportant, harmless things that you need to get rid of.

The National Association for Mental Health says there are a number of ways to tell if you are appropriately tense, or whether you might be reacting excessively. They suggest you ask yourself these questions:

• Do minor problems and disappointments throw you into a dither?

• Do you find it difficult to get along with people, and are people having trouble getting along with you?

• Do the small pleasures of life fail to satisfy you?

• Are you unable to stop thinking of your anxieties?

• Do you fear people or situations that never used to trouble you?

• Are you suspicious of people, mistrustful of your friends?

• Do you have the feeling of being trapped?

• Do you feel inadequate, suffer the tortures of self-doubt?

All of us will say yes to some of these questions, but if you answer yes to *most* of the questions, you may be suffering from excessive destructive anxiety and tension.

## What can you do to deal with your tensions?

If too much tension is a problem with you, what can you do about it?

The National Association for Mental Health makes these suggestions.

### 1. TALK IT OUT.

When something worries you, talk it out. Don't bottle it up. Confide your worry to some level-headed person you can trust: your husband or wife, father or mother, a good friend, your clergyman, your family doctor, a teacher, school counselor, or dean. Talking things out helps to relieve your strain, helps you to see your worry in a clearer light, and often helps you to see what you can do about it.

### 2. ESCAPE FOR A WHILE.

Sometimes, when things go wrong, it helps to escape from the painful problem for a while: to lose yourself in a movie or a book or a game, or take a brief trip for a change of scene. Making yourself "stand there and suffer" is a form of self-punishment, not a way to solve a problem. It is perfectly realistic and healthy to escape punishment long enough to recover breath and balance. But be prepared to come back and deal with your difficulty when you are more composed, and when you and others involved are in better condition to deal with it.

### 3. WORK OFF YOUR ANGER.

If you feel yourself using anger as a general way of behavior, remember that while anger may give you a temporary sense of righteousness, or even of power, it will generally leave you feeling foolish and sorry in the end. If you feel like lashing out at someone who has provoked you, try holding off that impulse for a while. Let it wait until tomorrow. Meanwhile, do something constructive with the pent-up energy. Pitch into some physical activity like gardening, cleaning out the garage, carpentry, or some other do-it-yourself project. Or work it out in tennis or a long walk. Working the anger out of your system and cooling it off for a day or two will leave you much better prepared to handle your problem.

### 4. GIVE IN OCCASIONALLY.

If you find yourself getting into frequent quarrels with people, and feeling obstinate and defiant, remember that that's the way frustrated children behave. Stand your ground on what you know is right, but do so calmly and make allowance for the fact that you could turn out to be wrong. And even if you're dead right, it's easier on your system to give in once in a while. If you yield, you'll usually find that others will, too. And if you can work this out, the result will be relief from tension, the achievement of a practical solution, together with a great feeling of satisfaction and maturity.

### 5. DO SOMETHING FOR OTHERS.

If you feel yourself worrying about yourself all the time, try doing something for somebody else. You'll find this will take the steam out of your own worries and—even better—give you a fine feeling of having done well.

## 6. Take one thing at a time.

For people under tension, an ordinary work load can sometimes seem unbearable. The load looks so great that it becomes painful to tackle any part of it—even the things that most need to be done. When that happens, remember that it's a temporary condition and that you can work your way out of it. The surest way to do this is to take a few of the most urgent tasks and pitch into them, one at a time, setting aside all the rest for the time being. Once you dispose of these you'll see that the remainder is not such a "horrible mess" after all. You'll be in the swing of things, and the rest of the tasks will go much more easily. If you feel you can't set anything aside to tackle things this sensible way, reflect: Are you sure you aren't overestimating the importance of the things you do—that is, your own importance?

## 7. Shun the "Superman" urge.

Some people expect too much from themselves, and get into a constant state of worry and anxiety because they think they are not achieving as much as they should. They try for perfection in everything. Admirable as this ideal is, it is an open invitation to failure. No one can be perfect in everything. Decide which things you do well, and then put your major effort into these. They are apt to be the things you like to do and, hence, those that give you most satisfaction. Then, perhaps, come the things you can't do so well. Give them the best of your effort and ability, but don't take yourself to task if you can't achieve the impossible.

## 8. Go easy with your criticism.

Some people expect too much of others, and then feel frustrated, let down, disappointed, even "trapped" when another person does not measure up. The "other person" may be a wife, a husband, or a child whom we are trying to fit into a preconceived pattern—perhaps even trying to make over to suit ourselves. Remember, each person has his own virtues, his own shortcomings, his own value, his own right to develop as an individual. People who feel let down by the shortcomings (real or imagined) of their relatives are really let down down about themselves. Instead of being critical about the other person's behavior, search out his good points and help him to develop them. This will give both of you satisfaction and help you to gain a better perspective on yourself as well.

9. GIVE THE OTHER FELLOW A BREAK.

When people are under emotional tension, they often feel that they have to "get there first"—to edge out the other person, no matter whether the goal is as trivial as getting ahead on the highway. If enough of us feel that way—and many of us do—then everything becomes a race in which somebody is bound to get injured—physically, as on the highway, or emotionally and mentally, in the endeavor to live a full life. It need not be this way. Competition is contagious, but so is cooperation. When you give the other fellow a break, you very often make things easier for yourself; if he no longer feels you are a threat to him, he stops being a threat to you.

10. MAKE YOURSELF "AVAILABLE."

Many of us have the feeling that we are being "left out," slighted, neglected, rejected. Often, we just imagine that other people feel this way about us, when in reality they are eager for us to make the first move. It may be we, not the others, who are deprecating ourselves. Instead of shrinking away and withdrawing, it is much healthier, as well as more practical, to continue to "make yourself available," to make some of the overtures instead of always waiting to be asked. Of course, the opposite of withdrawal is equally futile: to push yourself forward on every occasion. This is often misinterpreted and may lead to real rejection. There is a middle ground. Try it.

11. SCHEDULE YOUR RECREATION.

Many people drive themselves so hard that they allow themselves too little time for recreation—an essential for good physical and mental health. They find it hard to make themselves take time out. For such people, a set routine and schedule will help—a program of definite hours when they will engage in some recreation. And in general it is desirable for almost everyone to have a hobby that absorbs him in off hours—one into which he can throw himself completely and with pleasure, forgetting all about his work.

## Can you tell when stress is affecting your body?

Yes, there are many subliminal cues you can learn to recognize: gritting your teeth, tense forehead muscles, eyestrain, fluttering your eyelids, tension of neck muscles, irregular shallow breathing, cold hands, curled toes or fingers, butterflies in the solar plexus, voice stress, and increased pulse. When you feel them coming on, you can try consciously to relax them.

## Learning to relax

It's a lot easier to say, "Oh, relax and quit worrying so much," than it is to do it. But sometimes simply becoming aware of your over-tense state can be enough, so that you can talk to yourself and make yourself relax. Just saying, "Whoa, baby, take it easy," to yourself, stopping right there, taking two very deep breaths and going limp all over will often do the trick. Hard physical exercise is a great relaxer and tension reducer, also.

If you feel you are very tense and anxious, overreacting too many times and in too many situations, and you cannot relax yourself in these ways, you may need to get extra help in methods of relaxation. Progressive muscular relaxation, deep-breathing techniques, various yoga exercises and transcendental meditation have been of great benefit to many people. Especially when done on a regular basis, they help a person to naturally achieve a state of relaxation and inner calm that carries over into everyday activities. A number of scientific studies have shown that these methods can truly reduce tensions and anxieties and irritability and give one a new outlook on life and its problems.

One yogic exercise, called *shavasan*, has been used successfully in the management of hypertension by K. K. Datey, M.D., professor of medicine at the Medical College of Bombay. He reported on use of the technique in the medical journal *Angiology*, saying that, at first, patients came in every day to learn the exercise, then came in once a week to check their exercise technique and their blood pressures. Patients who were taking drugs were able in half the cases to reduce the dosage of the drugs by two-thirds, Dr. Datey said. But in those who did not do the exercise *regularly*, the drug doses could not be reduced.

Here in Dr. Datey's own words is a description of *shavasan*.

"The patient lies in the supine [on his back] position, lower limbs thirty degrees apart and the upper making an angle of fifteen degrees with the trunk, with the forearms in the midprone position and fingers semiflexed. The eyes are closed with eyelids drooping. The patient is taught slow rhythmic diaphragmatic breathing with a short pause after each inspiration and a longer one at the end of each expiration. After establishing this rhythm, he is asked to attend to the sensation at the nostrils, the coolness of the inspired air and the warmth of the expired air. This procedure helps to keep the patient inwardly alert and to forget his usual thoughts, thus becoming less conscious of external environment, thereby attaining relaxation. The patient is asked to relax the muscles so that he is able to feel the heaviness of different parts of the body. This is achieved automatically once the patient learns the exercise. The exercise is performed for thirty minutes. An experienced supervisor checks that there is no movement of any part of the body, except rhythmic abdominal movements.''

Classes in most of these techniques are available in major cities. Check with a psychologist, your doctor, a minister or priest, or a local health center.

### *Mind control through biofeedback*

Yogis have been known for years to be able to lower their blood pressure, slow down or speed up their heart rate, direct blood to circulate in one part of the body instead of another. Now research scientists have come up with a machine that helps a person to learn some of these same controls of the autonomic functions of their body. Continuous recordings are made of the function being studied, such as muscle tension, skin temperature or blood pressure, and a meter, a sound, or a flashing light tells the person whether he is getting the desired effect.

Control over these supposedly automatic functions was first shown in animals. Dr. Neal Miller of Rockefeller University showed that rats could raise or lower their blood pressure in response to rewards for such behavior. In fact, they could be trained to increase circulation to one ear and not the other and to increase blood flow to the kidneys which increased urine volume. Now this fascinating work has been extended to humans by Dr. Miller and by Drs. Lawrence D. Slotkoff at Georgetown University, David Shapiro at Harvard University, and Alvin Shapiro (no relation) at the University of Pittsburgh, all of whom have shown that man can also raise or lower his blood pressure at will. In a ninety-minute session two or three times a week, subjects are hooked up to a machine which sounds a tone when the blood pressure drops. So far, it is not known whether the effects will be long term, or whether the technique will have any real therapeutic value, but in the meantime it does indicate that our minds have some effect on our blood pressures.

With present techniques, most people have been able to produce changes of about 10 to 15 mm Hg in their pressure, although some have produced greater changes.

Apparently, if you are tense about it the technique doesn't work. It works best when the person is detached and passive and imagines the change in a calm and relaxed way. As researcher in the field, Dr. Elmer E. Green of the Menninger foundation says: "The idea is to *visualize, imagine,* and *feel* that the change is happening—and then just 'let it happen.'"

Says Dr. Green, "While using any kind of biofeedback device as a tool for learning something about yourself, it is interesting and instructive to experimentally induce in yourself a feeling of anxiety and nervousness, then calmness and tranquility. You can play with anger and with peacefulness. Then you can experiment with muscle tension, relaxation, slow deep breathing, etc. Learning to manipulate physiological processes while seeing the meter (or listening to it if it has an auditory output) is quite similar to learning to play a pinball machine."

The biofeedback technique is also being used with promising results to treat migraine headaches and cardiac arrhythmias, to ease tensions and produce general relaxation and self-awareness.

### Stress isn't all that bad

This doesn't mean we should try to avoid all stress in the world. Stress can add to the spice of life if it's not experienced in too-big doses. To have no stress at all would leave us no challenges, no goals, and life would be a vacuum of no runs, no hits, no errors.

All of us experience stress in life. Some people seem able to handle it better than others.

How can you improve the way you handle stress?

Read over again the suggestions from the National Association for Mental Health and see if some of those ideas might work for you. If you are in a period of particularly bad stress, try to interrupt it with some distraction like a movie, a swim, a walk, a game of tennis, a night of jazz.

If your deadline is tight and you simply cannot take time out, then try to keep from panicking by breaking down the job into steps and attacking them one at a time. Do your absolute best, and having done so, refuse to become anxious.

Or take the problem and analyze it on paper: what the problem really is, what your real goal is, what alternative answers are possible, the advantages and disadvantages of each. Many people find it helpful to study such a list before falling asleep, letting their brains work on it in a relaxed state through the night. Often our sleeping brains will see things in a new light, will realize that the logical solution isn't always the best. Sometimes we need to listen to our hearts. Or sometimes an hour of thinking on the seashore will make it a clear day when you can see, if not forever, at least the best possible way to act upon a problem.

Dr. Hans Selye, the world expert on stress, says that "the best way to avoid stress is to select an environment (wife, boss, social group) which is in line with our innate preferences, and to find an activity which we like and respect."

He tells how, when he got into medical school at the young age of eighteen, he was so fascinated by the possibilities of research on life and disease that he would get up at four in the morning to study. "I remember my mother telling me that this way of life could not be kept up for more than a couple of months, and would undoubtedly precipitate a nervous breakdown." Dr. Selye goes on to say, "Now I am sixty-six. I still get up at four o'clock in the morning and still work until six at night; yet I am perfectly happy leading this kind of life."

The only change he has made, he says, is to set aside an hour a day now to race around the McGill University campus on a bicycle between four and five in the morning "to combat the physical decay of senility."

If you really like what you are doing, if you love the person you are living with, then everyday problems can be handled. If your home and your job are giving you censure instead of approval, churning frustration instead of fulfillment and satisfaction, then think about ways you can change the situation in your world.

One thing to be on the lookout for is stress fatigue. When a person is in a period of emotional stress, he often lets himself become fatigued. Stress and fatigue together can be factors in triggering a heart attack. If you are in a period of stress, try to protect yourself by not adding on excessive fatigue.

# 14

# *Living with High Blood Pressure*

Once, there was a huge tidal wave on its way to Hilo, Hawaii. It was ten hours away. Hour after hour, radio announcements said it would arrive at midnight, warning the people to go to higher ground. Sirens sounded, and yet hundreds of people remained where they were. In the morning most of them were injured in the five hundred buildings washed away, and sixty-one were dead.

Why did they not act?

Why do people not see their doctors when they feel a lump or cough up blood? Why do seat belts lie unfastened; why do people keep smoking? Why do parents not take their children in for immunizations? Why, in an age when the art and science of medicine have reached such high development, do thousands let themselves die needlessly by not taking medicine or following advice they know can save them?

We know some of the reasons.

To begin with, there's the Superman Syndrome. Apparently, some people think it a sign of strength to suffer without complaining, a sign of weakness to get sick. A close relative is Perfect Paul. He has a concept of self-perfection and always thinks of himself as strong, sturdy, healthy, vigorous, young, handsome, and sexually desirable. To be sick is a flaw in the perfection.

There's the Ostrich Syndrome. Stick your head in the sand, deny you're sick, and maybe it will go away.

There's the Scared-To-Death Syndrome. The person becomes so afraid that he mistakenly feels that nothing can check the course of his illness or save his life. Or perhaps he or she is afraid of doctors and hospitals.

There's Fatalist Freddie, who says whatever will be, will be. And if the pink pill to cure his disease was lying on the floor in front of him, he wouldn't stoop over to pick it up.

There's the Poor-Little-Me Syndrome. Because you like the attention and sympathy, you figure it's kind of nice to be a little sick and you lean on it.

And there's the Fairy Godmother Syndrome. If you wait long enough, some miraculous cure will come along and make it all right again.

It's natural to have some resistance to accepting a diagnosis of a serious illness. Nobody wants to admit that his body has something wrong with it.

But with a disease like high blood pressure, you can do something about it! It doesn't pay to play Superman, or Ostrich, or Poor-Little-Me.

I tell my patients, "Look, you have high blood pressure, but the important thing is it can be controlled, and the complications can be prevented. You needn't have a stroke, or a coronary or premature death. Just stick with the treatment. You may have high blood pressure, but it is 'fixable.' "

Or, as Dr. Ted Cooper tells his patients: "Sure, you're going to die of something someday anyway. We all are. But we want to make it at age seventy or so—after we've had a full and happy life!"

So don't worry about your high blood pressure, do something about it!

A heart attack or stroke or kidney failure isn't something

that strikes you out of the blue. It builds up slowly with every added risk factor. But you can *do* something about those risk factors. You can lose weight, and stop smoking, and cut down on salt, and cut down on cholesterol, and exercise more, and try to relax more. And most of all, you can take your medicine for high blood pressure to keep this—*the biggest risk factor of all*—under control.

Don't gamble with the odds. It's not a horse race. It's the length—and quality—of your life that are the stakes.

## You can lead a full life

The quality of life is something doctors don't often talk to their patients about. The point in living is how well you are going to *live*. You don't want to drag through life puffing along short of breath, feeling tired, half there, unable to do the things you want to do. That way, you are simply existing—not living.

Nothing is more tragic than the person with twenty years of life ahead of him who finds himself crippled with a chronic disease.

If you keep your blood pressure down now, you can lead a full life for your *entire* life, functioning, productive, active, and happy.

Taking a few pills and reducing other risk factors is a small price to pay for getting the freedom to enjoy a really full life.

When Bob L. walked into his doctor's office and learned he had high blood pressure, his future actually started looking brighter. Because then he learned what to do. And what he does—now—can have a major effect on his health in the years to come. Starting today, if he does what the doctor says, there is every reason to believe that his blood pressure can be controlled. If, on the other hand, he decides to follow his old habits and ignore advice, he is leaving himself wide open to serious illness.

He has every reason for looking ahead with optimism. He knows he has it. The rest is up to him.

## *Working with your doctor*

High blood pressure is usually a lifelong disease. If you have it, you will probably be taking lifelong treatment, which makes it especially important for you to find a doctor or a clinic you like and trust—one that you can identify with, that will motivate you to continue with your medicine and keep up your appointments and help you to have fewer fears about your blood pressure. Try to find a doctor you can talk to, or a doctor with a nurse you can talk to, so you always feel free to ask questions and get advice.

In return, be a cooperative patient. Play your part, and follow his instructions. Tell the truth about whether you take your medicine or not. Your doctor can't keep you well if you don't do what he says.

Be a patient patient during trials of new medicines or new dosages. Don't expect your doctor to pull the right drug by magic like a rabbit out of a hat. He *should* experiment and try different drugs so that he can find, by trial and experience, just what the best drug is for you. Usually, though, there's not much experimenting, since the majority of patients have mild high blood pressure and most of those patients respond well to a pill a day, e.g., a thiazide diuretic.

Don't try to please your doctor by telling him you feel well when you don't. Some people lie to their doctors when asked how they feel, as though to protect him and please him. He doesn't *need* to be protected or pleased.

And usually he isn't very good at mind reading, so you must be free in telling him everything. Tell him if you're bitchy in your premenstrual period, or if you're dizzy in the morning, or if you have diarrhea, or if your sex life has suddenly disappeared. It's the only way he can tailor your treatment to fit your special needs.

One final caution: If you have blood pressure over 105 diastolic and your physician tells you not to worry about it because it "isn't bothering you," find another doctor who will do something for you.

## The reluctant patient

The biggest tragedy in the entire field of high blood pressure is that 40 to 70 percent of patients don't stay with their treatment.

Sometimes the patients leave the doctor's office and don't bother to have their prescriptions filled. Sometimes they get the pills, but don't take them, or take them for a while and then quit. Or they find them too expensive.

Unfortunately, some patients simply do not understand instructions. Sometimes—and all too frequently—instructions are not even given. A prescription is given to the patient as an afterthought—on his way out of the office. They do not realize that they must *continue* to take pills, and so quit taking the medicine because they feel better, or have finished the prescription and think they are cured, or take it only when they need it or give it up because of side effects without ever realizing that their doctor could change the medicine or the dosage.

Or they decide that their high blood pressure was just a case of nerves. Or even worse, some stop taking medicines because their doctors tell them to.

None of the advances in therapy is going to be realized— strokes, congestive heart failure, heart attack, and renal failure are not going to be prevented—unless the patient remains under medical care and takes his medication.

Data from several studies demonstrate the magnitude of the dropout problem. In 1963, Dr. Joseph Wilber surveyed the problem in Baldwin County, Georgia, where eleven physicians permitted him to review their records of six hundred hypertensive patients. Sixty to 70 percent of patients were lost to follow-up within two to three months! Thinking that this might be peculiar to a small-county population, he recently conducted a similar study in Atlanta of records of one thousand g.p's and internists there. They were losing 50 percent of their patients within a matter of months.

### *Fighting the dropout problem*

We recently analyzed the reasons for the high dropout rate in clinics in inner-city Washington and found that patients failed to return, not because they were dumb or did not want to know what high blood pressure could do to them, but because they were treated like a herd of cattle. The average waiting time before seeing the doctor was four and a half hours; the average time spent with the doctor was seven minutes. They were examined by a different doctor on each occasion which prevented any continuing communication or a meaningful doctor-patient relationship. The doctor wrote a prescription and sent them to the pharmacy where they waited another two hours. A few wasted days such as these, being herded into one room and then into another and having none of their questions answered, and it is no wonder that they soon stopped taking pills and did not return to the clinic. Unfortunately for many of them, the next contact with medical care was in a hospital emergency room because of a stroke.

Having learned something from this analysis, we reorganized our hypertension clinic, using the patient's complaints as guidelines. Operating our clinic with emphasis on a personalized doctor-patient relationship ( a nurse or para-medical person could substitute for the doctor), and using a meaningful appointment system (scheduling the appointment for 8:15 A.M. on Monday rather than just on Monday morning), our dropout rate was reduced from 42 percent to 4 percent!

The patient was always seen by the same paramedical interviewer, who weighed the patient, recorded heart rate and blood pressure, and asked about any unusual symptoms or side effects since the last visit. Until the blood pressure reached normal limits, the patient was routinely referred to the physician for re-evaluation and change in therapy. Otherwise the paramedical assistant or the pharmacist acted as a health counsellor, encouraging the patient not to smoke if he was a smoker, furnishing him with literature, giving him dietary instructions. This arrangement not only saved the clinic money, but freed the doctor to undertake more challenging tasks, and made the patients much happier and more cooperative.

Dr. John Caldwell, of Henry Ford Hospital in Detroit, has decreased his dropout problem by starting classes for patients on the problems of high blood pressure, medications, diets, and long-term care. There are informal sessions with six to eight patients, plus their spouses, because it's important to educate both the patient and the spouse so that someone you care for can give you support in following treatment.

### *Why do I need to keep seeing my doctor; why can't I just continue my pills?*

For several reasons. One: to make sure that your blood pressure hasn't gone up further. If so, it could be causing damage. Two: to see if your blood pressure has gone *down*. If so, you might be able to switch to a milder drug or a smaller dosage of the one you're on. Three: there are certain tests that the doctor needs to do periodically. For example, a test should be run occasionally to check the levels of potassium and sugar and other chemicals to see if they are in proper balance, or whether your pills are putting them out of whack.

So keep your appointments.

Remember high blood pressure has no symptoms. You are going to the doctor or clinic and taking your pills to *stay* well.

### *Should I be worried?*

No, because it won't do any good. Furthermore, you don't have to go around with a long face and act like an invalid. You can still lead an active, happy life.

The important thing is to be glad you found out you have a problem so that now you can do something about it.

### *The most important thing of all to remember*

You know to lose weight, to lower cholesterol intake, to exercise. You know to cut down on salt and to stop smoking. You know to try to ease tensions and keep from getting overly upset about things. These are all important. Do them.

But the most important thing of all if your doctor has you taking medicine is to take that medicine every day *when*ever and *how*ever your doctor says. Without fail. No matter what. Every day. For a long time, for the rest of your life.

What goes up can come down. Including your blood pressure. And taking your pill every day is a small price to pay to keep your pressure down where it belongs.

### *Make medication a habit*

Taking pills at certain times of the day can be easy if you make it a habit. Take your medication with meals, for example. Or make the pills a part of your getting-up or going-to-bed routine, if that is when you should take them. After a little practice you won't even think about it. Another good idea is to put the entire day's pills out in the morning in one special place so you will be reminded to take them.

### A close watch

Be sure to keep all your medical appointments. Especially at first, your physician will need to keep close watch over your progress in reducing your blood pressure. He will also probably make changes in your medication as you go along to meet your individual requirements, which he can diagnose only over a period of time.

### High blood pressure in children

If you have high blood pressure, have the pressure checked in your children. It's likely to be high also.

In fact, all children from about age three or four on should have their blood pressures checked every year as part of their regular physical exam. High blood pressure may well have its beginnings in childhood. Unfortunately, many pediatricians do not take blood pressures. Make sure that yours does.

We don't have extensive data on children as yet, but a study of seven thousand children in a government survey in 1965 showed an average blood pressure of 110/66 in children aged 6 to 11. A diastolic pressure (bottom number) of 85 in anyone under age 18 should be considered as hypertension.

If your child has high blood pressure, be sure to have his

cholesterol level checked also. If parents have high cholesterol levels in the blood, their children also tend to have
high levels, and this puts an added risk on the child.

Children with severe high blood pressure, just as adults,
require early treatment, including dietary restrictions and
anti-hypertensive drug therapy. See that he takes his pills.
Keep his weight down. Cut his salt intake. And see that he
sees his family doctor regularly.

More testing is needed in the child with severely high
pressure than in the adult because there are frequently
underlying causes such as kidney disease, or adrenal or
other tumors. These can usually be cured by surgery.

### Taking readings at home

More and more doctors are having their patients take their
own blood pressure readings at home. It's convenient, it
gives an up-to-the-minute check on what's really happening
to your pressure, and it gives you a way to check what
specific activities or events do to your pressure. And you can
actually see for yourself how your medicines keep your
pressure down.

As we have said, some doctors are not in favor of home
readings, believing it will make people overconcerned with
their pressures or the readings may be inaccurate. Others
think it is great, giving the person reassurance when he sees
his pressure is down to normal and alerting him when it's
up and he should see his doctor.

Some doctors would like to see a sphygmomanometer in
every home, as common as the bathroom scale and
thermometer.

Dr. Harriet P. Dustan, of the Cleveland Clinic in Ohio,
has been having patients take their home measurements for
more than twenty years. Dr. Dustan advises her patients to
take their readings in the morning on awakening, and just
before retiring, making it a daily routine, like brushing

teeth. They write down the measurements and mail them in to her once a month.

One caution about home readings: If someone is doing it for you, make sure his hearing is good. Some 10 to 15 percent of people are deaf enough not to be able to hear the sounds of the pulse accurately.

One instrument is even available now that shows blood pressure levels by lighting up, so a stethescope is not required.

## *Keeping track of yourself*

If you have high blood pressure, you might find it helpful to make a chart that will give you a chance to record your blood pressure and follow its course.

Each time you take your blood pressure or have it taken, write in the date on the chart and the number for both your systolic pressure and diastolic pressure. After a number of visits for checkups, you can see by the chart whether your blood pressure is staying about the same, or whether it is going up or down. Remember 140/90 is the satisfactory pressure you would like to reach. A pressure of 120/80 is the ideal.

If you have high blood pressure and are taking medication, enter the kind of medicine you are taking on each date also, and you will be able to see the actual effect of the medication on the blood pressure.

On the same days that you chart your blood pressure, also write down what your weight is. Then with one easy glance at this record you will be able to see changes that are occurring in blood pressure and weight.

## *How much rest is needed?*

Unless the hypertensive patient also has severe heart or kidney disease, extra daily rest is not necessary. To some people, a daily rest and early-to-bed are constant reminders that they are ill, and often produce more mental turmoil, not less. If you are tired, go to bed early or take a nap. If you're not tired, do what you want.

## Going to the bathroom

Most high blood pressure medicines are designed to increase urine output and so get rid of salt. The really powerful ones can produce a huge output of urine in fifteen to twenty minutes.

So take your frequent trips to the bathroom with a sense of humor. It shows your medicine is working. Make a bathroom stop before leaving the house, and if you use the pills that act in fifteen minutes, take them at home, not before you are going on a long bus ride.

## Drowsiness

Some pills can make you drowsy. Don't drive if you're drowsy, or work with dangerous tools.

## Getting out of bed

If you're the leap-out-of-bed-at-the first-click-of-the alarm-clock type, you may find yourself getting dizzy when you jump up, even to the point of passing out about the time you reach the bathroom. Don't panic. Simply get up more slowly. Sit up in bed. Dangle your feet over the side for a minute. Stand next to the bed a while in case you feel dizzy.

Also be careful about standing up suddenly out of a hot bathtub. Any time you feel faint, sit down.

If you have dizzy spells during the day, try wearing elastic support stockings.

These fainting spells, if they occur, are usually in the first days of starting the medicine or if doses are too high. If the problem continues, check with your doctor.

## Seasonal changes

The time of year can sometimes affect anti-hypertensive medication. For example, the dosage of diuretics can sometimes be reduced in patients during a hot summer, because increased perspiration removes extra salt from the system. But the dosage must be increased again during fall and winter.

In hot weather, by the way, don't drink too much water. And never take salt pills.

## High blood pressure and sex

If you have only mild high blood pressure, or your pressure is under good control with medicine, your sex life should not suffer at all. You can do everything as before.

If you have severe high blood pressure, or if the high blood pressure has caused heart damage or other complications, you should check with your doctor to see what he feels you can or cannot do sexually. There are a number of positions (such as the side position) which require less exertion than some of the others. It is not orgasm itself that causes increased pressure, but the exertion one can sometimes use to achieve it.

How your blood pressure reacts during sex can vary a great deal depending on how athletically you perform, as well as where you are and with whom. Heart attacks that occur during sexual intercourse are said to occur almost always during or after secret encounters when the person is not relaxed or is afraid of discovery.

For the couple accustomed to each other, sexual activity

is estimated to be about the same in exertion as climbing two flights of stairs or taking a fast walk. If you have no difficulty doing that, then sexual intercourse should give you no trouble.

One general rule for the patient with *severe* high blood pressure is not to do anything that causes distension of the neck veins. That would include lifting heavy things, straining at a bowel movement, or engaging in very strenuous intercourse. For the person on pills who has his pressure under control, any activity is okay.

### Impotence

Sid C. found that high blood pressure, because of its effect on his circulatory system, caused decreased interest in sex, and sometimes even impotence. Treating his high blood pressure brought sexual ability back again. On the other hand, some people find their high blood pressure pills cause impotence as a side effect. If this happens, discuss it with your physician, so he may prescribe a different pill.

Some pills, while not affecting orgasm, do have the strange effect of preventing ejaculation. This is not harmful in any way, and it is perfectly all right to continue sex and enjoy it for orgasm alone.

### Getting the blues

You are bound to get discouraged once in a while at having high blood pressure and needing to take pills all the time. Don't let it get you down. Be glad you know you have it so you can do something about it. Think about the people heading for trouble because they don't know about it.

If you become very depressed, really withdrawn, listless, and self-pitying, be sure to tell your doctor. Some medicines can cause depression and if yours is doing this he will want to give you a different kind.

Do what your doctor tells you, but don't get so overly concerned about your blood pressure that you turn into a hypochondriac. Unless you already have some secondary damage to your heart or kidneys, your life need not be different than it was before.

### Are there any warning signs or symptoms I should be on the lookout for?

Yes. Don't go around staring at yourself in the mirror all day. People will think you are a hypochondriac. But if you have any new symptoms, or resurgence of old ones, do call your doctor and let him know. He may be unconcerned and tell you not to worry. Or he may want you to come in for a readjustment of medicine or some different treatment.

Chances are, if you take your pills as your doctor directs, everything will be fine. Occasionally, warning signs of danger do occur.

Here are the times when you should call your doctor for an appointment:

If your tissues are swollen or soggy from fluid accumulation. You can spot accumulation in tissues if you are alert for such things as difficulty in getting into your shoes (swollen feet) or difficulty in getting rings on and off. In fact, we even use jeweler's ring sizers to test patients for swollen fingers at regular checkups.

Other signs of water buildup are sudden weight gain with no change in diet, puffiness of the face, rings under the eyes, swollen ankles or feet, or a feeling of being bloated and waterlogged. You should buy a bathroom scale if you don't already have one. Weigh yourself daily at the same time every day. Any gain of weight of over two pounds means fluid retention.

If you have difficulty in breathing. You should check with your doctor if you repeatedly have to be propped up to breathe easily in bed, if you wake up wheezing or short of breath in the middle of the night, or if you have shortness of breath when you climb a flight of stairs or hurry for a bus.

You should check with your doctor if you have frequent muscle cramps or if you ever have to stop walking because of pains in your legs.

These latter symptoms are most commonly caused by a decrease in the content of potassium—due to excess loss in the urine—which is due to the diuretic. It is readily correctable by adding another pill or a potassium supplement.

### When to act immediately

If you ever have signs of a heart attack or stroke, you should call your doctor *immediately*.

Sometimes symptoms subside, then return. When you experience one or more warning signs, call your doctor and describe these symptoms in detail. If he's not immediately available, get to a hospital emergency room at once.

Be prepared to act! Instruct others to act if you cannot. Keep a list of numbers—doctor, hospital, ambulance or other emergency services and police—next to your telephone, and in a prominent place in your pocket, wallet, or purse.

### The warning signs of heart attack

Prolonged, heavy pressure or a squeezing pain in the center of the chest, behind the breastbone.

Pain may spread to the shoulder, arm, neck, or jaw.

Pain or discomfort is often accompanied by sweating.

Nausea, vomiting, and shortness of breath may also occur.

The pain of a heart attack or "angina" is never sharp like a knife. It is usually not over the heart and is not made worse by deep breathing. A sharp pain over the right or left side of your chest, therefore, is not indicative of a heart attack, particularly if it is made worse by taking a deep breath or a certain motion.

### *The warning signs of stroke*

Sudden, temporary weakness or numbness of the face, arm, or leg.

Temporary difficulty or loss of speech, or trouble understanding speech.

Temporary dimness or loss of vision, particularly in one eye.

An episode of double vision.

Unexplained dizziness or unsteadiness.

Change in personality, mental ability, or pattern of headaches.

Sometimes strokes occur as "little strokes," so temporary you may not even realize that you have had one.

Little strokes—or, in medical parlance, cerebral transient ischemic attacks (TIAs)—are characterized by such symptoms as momentary numbness or weakness of an arm or leg, headaches, abrupt clumsiness (jerky handwriting, for example), temporary loss of vision, or short memory lapses. And, although they may only last two minutes or so, they often are a signal that a full-fledged stroke is in the offing, though it may be days, weeks or months away.

If a person has a stroke and is then discovered for the first time to have high blood pressure, the pressure needs to be treated, but should be lowered gradually rather than suddenly. Lowering the blood pressure is the most important thing you can do to prevent occurrence of another stroke. The better you control your high blood pressure, the less likely you are to ever have another stroke.

## Hypertensive emergencies

An acute hypertensive crisis where the blood pressure goes shooting up to dangerous heights can sometimes happen in high blood pressure, particularly if patients do not keep up with their medication.

Warning signs of an impending crisis are severe headache caused by the sudden elevation of pressure, dizziness or difficulty with vision. There also may be difficulty in breathing, or bleeding from the nose.

The person should go to the hospital. In a few instances, if the person does not get treatment, there may be convulsions, coma, or stroke.

In the hospital, a number of medicines are available for quick and effective treatment, especially the new drugs diazoxide and furosemide. They work in one or two minutes, reducing the blood pressure by as much as one-third.

These emergencies happen rarely now that there are effective drugs. If you take your pills regularly and keep in touch with your doctor, the chances are slight that you will ever have such an experience.

## Once damage is done, is it too late?

Absolutely not. The thing to do is correct what can be corrected and prevent further damage from being done. But if some damage has been done already, it is doubly important that you follow your doctor's advice, always taking your pills regularly and carrying out other orders.

This is no time to play around with a blasé attitude of knowing more than your doctor.

Take your pills, all of them, on time, whenever you should.

Report all symptoms and signs to your physician, right away, so he can determine if they are significant in any way.

Keep your appointments. It is important that your doctor should keep close tabs on you so he can pick up any changes in your blood pressure or vital functions, always being on top of things as they are first happening—when they can more easily be fixed.

### *If you get sick and have a fever*

Sometimes when you have a fever, you get side effects from your pills when you never had them before. This is because fever for some reason seems to reduce the dosage requirements you need. If you are ill with a high fever, check it out with your doctor.

### *If you are going to have surgery*

Since blood pressure shouldn't be abnormally low or the chemicals in your body unbalanced during surgery, blood pressure medicines are usually stopped about two weeks before surgery is scheduled. Your doctor will tell you when to start up again.

If you have to go for emergency surgery at any time, be sure to tell the surgeon and the anesthetist that you are on medicine for high blood pressure so they can take that into account in planning the anesthesia and other procedures related to surgery.

### Can a person with high blood pressure donate blood?

If you have written permission from your physician, most blood banks will accept a donor whose diastolic pressure is no higher than 110. However, without special permission, they ordinarily will refuse you as a donor if your pressure is higher than 100 diastolic.

### Taking other medicines

Some drugs, like oil and water, just don't mix. And when you take them together they can cause side effects; one drug can make the other one more powerful, or can cut down its effect; or a whole new set of symptoms can be caused. The interactions of drugs are so complex and so potentially serious that one medical writer, Dr. Eric Martin, has written an entire book simply listing drugs and their interactions.

For example, Mary T. was taking the high blood pressure drug guanethidine. It was doing fine for her, holding her blood pressure down with no side effects. Then suddenly on the next checkup the doctor found Mary's blood pressure back up again. After much examining and questioning he learned that Mary had been taking an amphetamine as an appetite suppressant to try to lose weight—without telling him. As soon as he took her off the appetite drug, the guanethidine worked fine again.

The high blood pressure drugs you take can have an effect on other medicines, too. If you are taking digitalis for a heart condition, taking a thiazide for your high blood pressure can drastically change the amount of digitalis you need.

You shouldn't take any other drugs, even ones you can buy over the counter yourself in the drugstore, without first checking with your physician. And when your physician gives you instructions on your high blood pressure medicine, be sure that the instructions are written down, and follow them to the letter. Don't increase or decrease the dosage yourself, only do it if he specifically tells you to.

Also, always be sure to tell your doctor about any other health problems you might have. Certain high blood pressure medicines can aggravate ulcers, asthma, gout, or depression. Some medicines can be used if you have congestive heart failure, or have had a heart attack or stroke. Some cannot. Some can be used when there is kidney damage, some cannot.

## *If you have glaucoma*

Glaucoma affects the pressure within your eyeball. If you have it, be sure to tell your doctor because he will then want to lower your blood pressure more gradually. Since the eye is accustomed to the high pressure of glaucoma, it needs time to adjust to new pressures and too rapid a change can cause damage.

## *If you have diabetes*

There seems to be some relationship between diabetes and high blood pressure, but doctors do not really understand at this time what the tie-in is. They do know that people with diabetes are somewhat more likely to have high blood pressure than persons who do not have diabetes.

If you are taking insulin, you may have to work with your doctor in adjusting the dosage of the insulin because the requirements are frequently changed by high blood pressure medicine. Strangely, sometimes more insulin is needed, sometimes less, and sometimes there is no change in requirements.

Sometimes, latent diabetes that the person did not even

know he had will come to the fore and start showing signs after the person has been on high blood pressure medicine for a while. We don't know why.

The important thing to know about having high blood pressure *and* diabetes is that they both cause damage to the circulation, so that you are in double jeopardy. It is an extra risk factor that makes it doubly important to follow advice and take your medicines for both conditions.

## *Hypertension and birth control pills*

There are three periods in life when women seem to have the most trouble with high blood pressure: On birth control pills, during menopause (or when ovaries are removed by surgery), and during pregnancy.

High blood pressure is a very rare side effect of birth control pills when one considers the many millions of women who show only very slight or no pressure reaction at all. But in some women, the pills do seem to bring on high pressure. It seems to be the old story of predisposition.

One recent survey of six hundred women in inner-city Washington who were taking birth control pills showed that 7 percent who had no history of an elevated blood pressure developed high blood pressure while taking the pill. Of patients who had a history of an elevated blood pressure prior to taking the pill, 7 percent had worsening of their blood pressure while taking the pill. The incidence of pill-induced hypertension in other studies ranges between 3 and 17 percent.

How many of these women would have developed high blood pressure anyway is not known.

With the women in our clinic who have high blood pressure and are taking a birth control pill, we have them stop taking the pill and use another contraceptive, and follow their blood pressure closely for three months. If their pressure is lowered at all when away from the birth control pill, then they stay off birth control pills permanently and use other methods of contraception.

On the other hand, if the blood pressure does not come down, then the birth control pill can be continued, if indicated, and anti-hypertensive medication instituted.

The risk of having a stroke is higher in women who take birth control pills, too. But the rate of stroke with pills is lower than the rate with pregnancy, and even with the increased risk, the actual number of strokes that occur is small.

Whether you have normal pressure or high pressure, if you take birth control pills or take hormone pills for any reason, you should be doubly sure to have regular periodic checks of your blood pressure. If you are just starting on birth control pills, you should have your blood pressure checked about every two months for the first year.

### Danger during menopause

Two things happen during menopause. Your estrogen levels go down and the amounts of pituitary hormones go up. Both of these hormone changes can affect the blood vessels and the blood pressure; and the changes, in fact, are held responsible for the great increase in the number of strokes and heart attacks that occur in women after menopause.

From the beginning of menopause on, you should be sure that your gynecologist takes your blood pressure and tells you what it is. Most gynecologists now also do vaginal smears for estrogen levels at the same time they do a Papanicolau smear. If your estrogen levels are low, many gynecologists believe you should take estrogen pills. The estrogen eliminates most of the symptoms of menopause, helps prevent osteoporosis of the bones that occurs in later life, and improves the lubrication and tone of the vaginal tract. The pills are taken for twenty-five days each month and stopped for five days to simulate the natural hormone cycle. But estrogen can also cause an instability of the circulatory systems, so you should have your blood pressure checked regularly if you start on the pills.

The estrogen changes in menopause usually take two or three years. If ovaries are removed surgically, the hormone level drops immediately and sharply so that menopause symptoms are severe and make the woman very uncomfortable. Usually women with "surgical menopause" are started on estrogen replacement immediately before even leaving the hospital.

Estrogen, by the way, is produced in the adrenal glands and liver as well as by the ovaries, but the levels are small and cannot substitute for the large amounts produced by the ovaries.

## *Pregnancies and high blood pressure*

Blood pressure may go up in pregnancy, go down, or stay the same. Your pressure may have been normal before and suddenly goes high for the first time in your life. Or you may have had high blood pressure before you were pregnant and now it becomes normal. Or it may go up after delivery for several weeks or months, then drop to normal. High blood pressure, however, greatly increases the chances of your developing toxemia, i.e., your chances now are 66 to 1. Developing toxemia is bad because it not only has an effect on your blood pressure and kidneys but also on the fate of the baby, increasing the risk of your baby's being born prematurely or dead.

If you have high blood pressure and you become pregnant, get in touch with your doctor right away because he may want to make some adjustments in your medication. Some high blood pressure medicines, for example, cross the placenta and so would affect the developing embryo. Others do not.

Also be sure to tell your obstetrician that you have high

blood pressure and are taking medicines for it. He and your other doctor may want to keep in touch on your medical care during pregnancy.

Usually, if you have been taking high blood pressure medicine before pregnancy, you should continue taking it during pregnancy.

If you have high blood pressure during pregnancy, you may be likely to have high pressure also when taking contraceptive pills. Be sure to discuss this with your obstetrician as well as your regular doctor.

### Toxemia

High blood pressure can be a sign of toxemia, a disease that occurs—cause unknown—in a number of pregnancies.

In toxemia, the woman first gets retention of sodium with swelling of the hands and under the eyes. Later, there is high blood pressure and albumin in the urine. If treated successfully and early enough, pregnancy can continue. If untreated, the woman may go into convulsions and coma, and the pregnancy may have to be terminated.

As a check against toxemia every pregnant woman should see her doctor every month for the first six months for urinalysis and blood pressure check. In the seventh and eight months, checkups should be every two weeks; during the last month, every week.

### What about nursing if you are taking high blood pressure pills?

Thiazides and several of the other blood pressure pills do appear in breast milk when the mother takes it. If your high blood pressure is mild enough and you want to nurse your baby, talk over with your doctor whether you could stop your medicine for a short while, just through the nursing period. If he thinks your blood pressure is so high you should not stop taking the pills even for a short time, then you should not nurse your baby.

# 15

# Special Types of High Blood Pressure

Mary T. lived next door to us down at the lake. The thirty-year-old wife of a dentist, she was cute, vivacious, and sparkling, always ready for a game of tennis or a fling at the water skis. Then suddenly one summer she began having problems—headaches, really bad headaches, flashes of sweating, palpitations of the heart. She went to the doctor and found a scary pressure of 180/120. Nothing seemed to bring it down. She walked through a day as if she were on eggshells, afraid that the slightest exertion might be enough to burst a blood vessel straining from the high pressure. The doctor ran a series of tests and found it was a tiny tumor called a pheochromocytoma, located in her abdomen. She went to a medical center, had the tumor removed, and today is as good as new.

Mary was one of the people in the 10 percent, the ones who do not have essential hypertension with cause unknown, but who have a kind of hypertension in which the cause can be found and can be cured.

The causes can be many things: A pinching of a main artery coming from the chest, an abnormality of the kidneys, or a tumor that secretes hormones and chemicals that make the blood pressure rise.

Since the cause is known, in these cases a direct attack can be made by the doctor to cure them. Usually the answer is surgery—correcting the pinched artery, removing a diseased kidney, taking out a tumor. Sometimes certain medicines will do the trick, also.

The high blood pressure due to known causes is sometimes called secondary hypertension, that is, it is a secondary result of other problems.

More and more specific causes are being found for high blood pressure. So, as time goes on, a greater number of cases will be fixable with surgery.

### Clues to curable high blood pressure

The first hint that a curable form of high blood pressure may be present is when ordinary blood pressure medicines do not bring it down or when the medicines bring the pressure down at first, but it soon starts to go up again.

There are other clues, too. A curable form of high blood pressure with known cause often comes on suddenly. Essential high blood pressure often begins gradually. There is often a family history of essential high blood pressure. In the other forms, this factor is usually not present.

In pheochromocytoma, such as Mary T. had, there is often profuse sweating of the face and body.

In disease of the arteries of the kidney, there are often pains in the upper leg and blood in the urine.

Another kind of kidney problem would be indicated if the person had a history of urinary tract infections.

Frequent urination, including at night, and muscle weakness might indicate aldosteronism, one of the high blood pressure conditions caused by a tumor.

## Laboratory tests

Once the clues have pointed the way toward the possibility of one of the less common forms of high blood pressure, your doctor will do various tests to confirm just which condition is the cause in your particular case. For example, a high aldosterone level in the blood might indicate aldosteronism, and a high level of metanephrine in the urine might indicate pheochromocytoma.

These tests, as noted earlier, are not done in every case of high blood pressure, only when there is reason to believe one of the forms other than essential hypertension is present. Curable forms of high blood pressure are so rare it just isn't logical to subject all patients to costly, unnecessary tests.

The only exception to this might be in hypertension patients under age thirty-five, since the rare forms occur more frequently in this group than in patients over that age.

## Malignant hypertension (accelerated hypertension)

Malignant hypertension is not just bad hypertension, but is actually an entirely different disease, with eye and kidney symptoms, weight loss, and severe deterioration and inflammation of the blood vessels. The diastolic pressure is greater than 140, there are flame-shaped hemorrhages and swelling of the nerve head in back of the eyes. There is an actual breakdown of the arterioles, especially in the kidneys, and if it is untreated, death occurs usually in two years by kidney failure in 95 percent of people.

This form of hypertension can come on after a patient has had regular hypertension or, it can suddenly start up on its own, without any previous history of high blood pressure.

Malignant hypertension is so named not because of any relationship to cancer, but because of its previously highly fatal course. Similar to essential hypertension, its cause is not known.

The disease used to be considered nearly always fatal. This is no longer true and many patients with this form of hypertension today are alive to show that the disease is now considered reversible. But early treatment is imperative. The blood pressure must be controlled before kidney function has gone past the "point of no return."

J.C., a thirty-one-year-old black male, came to the clinic with a history of blurred vision, severe headache, and a weight loss of twenty pounds in the past month. Interesting was the fact that he had been to a private doctor who apparently did not even take his blood pressure, but sent him for stomach x-rays, thinking that he must have cancer because of the weight loss.

Physical examination revealed his blood pressure to be 220/140 mm Hg. Examination of the back of his eyes showed that the blood vessels had ruptured, which accounted for his blurred vision. The remainder of the examination was fairly unremarkable except for enlargement of his heart.

He was hospitalized and treated just as though he had a hypertensive emergency, i.e., he received intravenous diazoxide to control his blood pressure continuously over a two-week period, and a potent diuretic to maintain the output of urine. An hour after his blood pressure had been lowered, his headaches disappeared, and in four days the blurred vision began to clear. By the time of discharge, two weeks later, he was able to read the newspaper.

He was sent home on oral anti-hypertensives and a diuretic. From that time on, he was seen at monthly intervals.

When seen most recently, his blood pressure was 130/80 mm Hg, and he had been working every day.

The key to treatment is to keep the pressure down as low as possible and maintain the output of urine, thus preventing further damage or stroke, while the arterioles have a chance to heal from their strange inflammation. To do this, the high blood pressure is treated as an emergency and the patient put in the hospital so that the doctor can bring the blood pressure down rapidly and aggressively.

The two drugs used most to reduce the blood pressure and keep it down, and to maintain the output of urine, are diazoxide, given by injection into the vein, and furosemide, given intravenously or orally. Because the disease is so dangerous and the results of treatment so good, we believe emergency treatment should begin immediately as soon as the diagnosis is made. Investigations to determine the cause of the disease can be done after the pressure has been brought under control. The imminent danger of a stroke in these patients is so high that safety demands emergency treatment. The newer, more powerful drugs currently available in Europe may improve the prognosis of these patients even more.

### Coarctation of the aorta

The aorta is an artery that's as big as a garden hose, coming directly from the heart to take blood to the body. In some people this artery is constricted at birth.

It's an easy condition to spot. The doctor takes the blood pressure in the arms, finds it high. Then he takes a pressure reading at a leg artery and finds it much lower. He has you jump up and down until you're out of breath, then measures the pressure again. If there is coarctation (constriction) of the aorta, the pressure in the arm arteries may have skyrocketed to some 300 mm Hg systolic.

Sometimes the constriction is shown up by pulsating arteries in the back. And a chest x-ray may show telltale notching of the ribs.

Coarctation of the aorta is corrected by surgery. The surgeon simply puts clips on the aorta to stop the blood, cuts out the constricted part and sews the two ends back together again. If the constricted part is extensive, a dacron or teflon graft may be used to join up the two ends.

The blood pressure immediately goes down, right on the operating table, and after a couple of weeks in the hospital for recuperation, the patient usually goes home with perfectly normal pressure.

### *Pheochromocytoma*

Of all the high blood pressure diseases, pheochromocytoma is the best understood, the easiest to diagnose, and the surest to treat. This is the disease that Mary T. had—a tumor of the middle of the adrenal gland. The tumor can also occur around the nerves of the neck, chest, abdomen, and pelvis. But most are in the adrenal glands or in the abdomen.

The tumor can appear in early childhood or old age, but usually occurs in the forties. Occasionally it is cancerous, but most of the time not.

The symptoms vary greatly. Most commonly seen are those due to the outpouring of adrenalin, e.g., headaches, sweating, pounding heart, nausea, trembling, weakness, tiredness, nervousness, steady high blood pressure, occasional surges of high pressure that come and go, racing heart, and fever. The spells of high blood pressure may be brought on by exercise, bending over, urination, defecation, smoking, or pressure on the abdomen. The patient is sometimes brushed off as being a hypochondriac when he describes these spells of tightness starting in the abdomen and rising to the chest and head, tremors, sweating, and palpitations of the heart followed by extreme weakness. In truth, the blood pressure during one of these attacks may be as high as 250/105 mm. Hg or more!

Since 95 percent of patients with pheochromocytoma are thin, obesity greatly minimizes the chances of such symptoms being due to this type of a tumor. When a number of these clues indicate that the person may have pheochromocytoma, the doctor can confirm the diagnosis by a urine test.

More often than not the person turns out *not* to have the disease since it is often mimicked by periodic rises in blood pressure in patients with anxiety accompanied by labile hypertension. However, the urine test will show up the true condition.

The procedure usually is to remove the tumor by surgery. Treatment is absolutely necessary, and when done, usually gives instant relief. If not treated, the condition is almost always fatal. During the operation, the surgeon explores the entire abdomen for other possible tumors to make sure he has removed them all.

If a single tumor on one adrenal gland is found, the entire gland is removed. If there are tumors on both glands, some adrenal tissue is left so the patient does not have to have hormone replacement for life.

If for any reason surgery is not feasible, the condition can be treated medically.

Patients should also take medicines before surgery to control blood pressure and reduce risks from surgery due to the swings of pressure. The outlook for patients is usually excellent. If the tumors are completely removed, the blood pressure should be normal. But urine tests should be run every year for a few years just for assurance.

### Renal hypertension

Renal hypertension is the most common kind of high blood pressure where the cause is known. *Renal* refers to kidney. "Renal hypertension" is high blood pressure that is caused by some damage in the arteries leading to the kidney or in the kidneys themselves. Since one-fourth of the entire output of the heart goes to the kidneys, obstruction and resistance in the kidneys can cause a rise in pressure in the entire circulatory system. It has been estimated that 5 to 10 percent of all cases of hypertension may be due to kidney disease, and that there may be as many as two million undiagnosed cases of renal hypertension in the United States. With accurate diagnosis and treatment, many of these victims could be cured or substantially improved. It should be emphasized, however, that fully half of these patients respond well to usual medical therapy (taking pills) and probably an additional 25 percent should not be operated on because of other complications. The number of patients actually helped by surgery, therefore, is quite limited.

The kidney damage can be caused in two ways.

If there is damage to the arteries that go to the kidneys, providing blood, the hypertension is called *renovascular hypertension*. It can occur in both kidneys, but usually attacks one more than the other. Sometimes, especially over age fifty, the damage to the renal arteries is caused by fatty deposits on the artery walls from atherosclerosis narrowing the arteries.

Other conditions that narrow the arteries tend to occur in younger persons. Sometimes the narrowing can be in one small artery going to one part of one kidney and yet be enough to cause high blood pressure.

It is not easy to diagnose renal hypertension at first, but it may be suspected when there is a rather sudden onset of the high blood pressure or an abrupt worsening of high blood pressure that medicines don't help. It can also be suspected when the doctor hears a high pitched murmur with the stethoscope over the abdomen.

Final diagnosis is done by several tests. One test, called an intravenous pyelogram, involves injecting a dye into a vein in the arm and then watching through an x-ray machine as the dye works its way through the bloodstream and then circulates through the kidney, outlining the kidneys and sometimes the kidney arteries as it goes.

When renovascular hypertension is suspected, a dye is

injected directly into the artery in the groin and traced by serial x-rays as it passes through the kidney.

Demonstrating any abnormality—e.g., obstruction, calcium plaque, or narrowing of an artery—does not necessarily mean that this abnormality is the cause of the elevated blood pressure.

It must be proved that this abnormality is actually causing damage to the particular kidney and that the involved kidney is therefore pouring forth an excess of a substance which increases the blood pressure. This substance is called renin.

Having demonstrated an abnormality, then we must measure the amount of renin coming from each kidney. This can be done at the same time as the dye injection, thus not subjecting the patient to another unnecessary procedure. If the amount of renin coming from the diseased kidney is more than two and one-half times that coming from the other kidney, then that kidney or the artery leading to that kidney is the cause of the elevated blood pressure and, all things being equal, should be corrected by surgery. Administering a potent diuretic fifteen to twenty minutes prior to the collection of the renin sample has been shown to magnify the differences, thus making it easier to determine a positive result.

None of these tests is foolproof (sometimes they give false positive or false negative results), but together they can be most helpful.

Often renovascular hypertension can be treated medically with pills just as other types of high blood pressure. When this does not work, it can usually be cured by surgery. Sometimes the inside of the artery obstructed by fatty deposits is reamed out. Sometimes the diseased section of the artery is simply removed or another blood vessel is transplanted to the kidney. If a kidney is badly damaged, it may be completely removed, with the remaining kidney carrying on alone.

If both kidneys have to be removed, then kidney dialysis treatments may be necessary. It used to be that the person who needed dialysis had to go to the hospital two or three times a week, being hooked up to an artificial kidney machine for six or seven hours each time so that the machine could do the job of his kidneys, clearing the blood of chemicals and wastes, making it pure again. Now there are less expensive and simpler artificial kidney machines, so that dialysis can be done at home.

Kidney transplants can also be considered. Whether to have surgery or use medicines is something that you and your doctor will have to work out together, based on the advantages for your particular situation.

The second cause of kidney damage that can result in high blood pressure is the reaction of the kidney to a streptococcal infection. A typical case is that of a child with a streptococcal infection of the throat or impetigo which leads to an inflammation of the kidney called glomerulo-nephritis. You know the kidney has been affected when the child passes dark urine or develops swelling of the face. The condition can occur in children or adults. Sometimes the high blood pressure thus caused disappears as fast as it developed, but in other cases it lingers on and leads to chronic kidney disease and long-lasting high blood pressure. This kind of damage is identified by checking for abnormal proteins or white cells in the urine. The utmost care should be taken to prevent recurrences of streptococcal infection. For example, your physician will probably prescribe an antibiotic, particularly during the winter months, and will want to see you for sure whenever you should develop a throat or skin infection.

Repeated infections of the bladder or kidney can cause a third kind of renal hypertension. The repeated infections can lead to scarring of the kidney—frequently more on one side than the other. Such scarring may actually lead to the shrinking or shriveling of one kidney which may, in rare instances, cause high blood pressure. Removal of the shrunken kidney may result in a cure of the high blood pressure.

Another type of renal hypertension has been described by Dr. Jerome W. Conn and colleagues of the University of Michigan Medical School. They reported discovery of a tumor of the kidney that produces the enzyme renin to raise blood pressure. Five cases of the tumor have been reported so far, with the tumor tissue being found to contain twenty-seven times more renin than the kidney tissue around it.

When the kidney with the tumor was removed, all symptoms were gone within six days.

### *Aldosteronism*

It was only twenty years ago that excessive secretion of a hormone aldosterone from the kidney was discovered, also by Dr. Conn, to be a cause of high blood pressure. The excess hormone production can be caused by a little pea-sized tumor, or in children by abnormal kidney tissue.

The condition is rare, probably occurring in less than 1 percent of people with high blood pressure, but can occur at any age. About one thousand cases have been found since discovery of this disease, but some physicians believe that there are many cases that go unrecognized and could be cured.

In these cases, blood pressure can be moderate or high, but does not usually reach the dangerous peaks of some of the other rare high blood pressures. Colonel R. had the typical symptoms. He tired easily, and had muscle weakness, muscle twitchings, frequent urination day and night, and frequent thirst, prickling sensations, and headache. The first clue to the excess secretion of aldosteronism—which not everyone has—was muscle weakness that followed thiazide administration when his doctor first treated what he believed to be a simple case of high blood pressure. The second clue was when the colonel's urinalysis showed an alkaline rather than the usual acid urine, and his serum potassium levels were excessively low.

When the doctor recognized these clues, Colonel R. was referred to a medical center for further evaluation to establish a firm diagnosis of primary aldosteronism.

The tumors—adenomas—that usually are the cause of aldosteronism are small, maybe only an inch in diameter. They may occur on one or both kidneys, usually on the left one. They are not malignant.

The disease can sometimes be treated medically with a medicine called spironolactone. Or—as in the colonel's case—it may be treated surgically in a medical center by a physician experienced in adrenal surgery. When the tumors are removed, 95 percent of patients show improvement. The colonel's blood pressure dropped gradually and became normal several months after the operation.

Primary aldosteronism refers to excess secretion of the hormone from a tumor or tissue within the kidney.

Secondary aldosteronism refers to excess secretion of the hormone because of some factor outside the kidney which stimulates it to produce more of the hormone.

### Licorice-eaters

Eating a lot of licorice can produce a baffling kind of high blood pressure that closely resembles aldosteronism and many a doctor has been fooled by it. Who in the world would think to tell the doctor about their favorite kind of candy?

A chemical in licorice is converted to another chemical in the body that just happens to cause retention of sodium and so raises blood pressure.

One patient ate an average of a pound of licorice a week and had a blood pressure of 170/120. His laboratory tests all pointed toward a diagnosis of aldosteronism and it looked as though he might have to have surgery. When his licorice habit was discovered and stopped, blood pressure in two weeks dropped to 160/100, and in three months it was down to 140/92.

A medicine containing some of the same chemicals in licorice is used in England to treat ulcers and can produce the same high blood pressures as is found in licorice-eaters.

## Cushing's syndrome

High blood pressure is a problem in most patients with Cushing's syndrome, a hormone disease named after the man who first described it—Dr. Harvey Cushing. This disease, like primary aldosteronism, is due to excessive secretions of hormone from the kidneys, but this time the hormone is hydrocortisone. In addition to high blood pressure, the person begins to change in appearance, becoming thick in the body, round-faced, humped in the shoulders, and hairy.

Diagnosis is confirmed by laboratory tests.

Sometimes the disease is caused by a tumor of the adrenal gland, or of the pituitary gland. Treatment is surgical removal of the tumor, or if surgery is not possible, chemotherapy of the tumor is done. Sometimes an adrenal gland must be removed.

If a tumor is found and removed, the removal usually produces a gradual return of the patient's condition to normal.

## Pulmonary hypertension

If a patient suddenly has unexplained shortness of breath, or sudden heart failure, it can often be due to pulmonary hypertension, an increase in blood pressure due to blockage of blood vessels of the lungs by blood clots.

Sometimes, if the clots are small, the person might not notice the episode, but if more clots block more blood vessels, death can eventually occur.

But if the condition is caught in time, appropriate treatment can stop and even reverse the condition. Most patients with this kind of high blood pressure are age forty or over. Diagnosis is by x-ray and electrocardiogram.

Part of the treatment is to take anticoagulant medicine to prevent further clots from forming. Special medicines are also used to try to dissolve the clots. Sometimes surgery is necessary.

### Other causes

A number of other conditions can cause high blood pressure.

High pressure occurs when there are extensive burns over the body or after several kinds of heart surgery, but these are temporary forms of hypertension.

High pressure also can occur with brain tumors, with thyroid diseases, with spinal cord injuries, with syphilitic crises, and with poliomyelitis.

Patients with aortic aneurysms—those balloon-like weaknesses of the main artery from the heart—often have high pressure also. Because the thin walls of the aneurysm are likely to rupture, it has been considered essential that the aorta be repaired by immediate surgery. But getting the blood pressure down to normal can often be a life-saving measure in itself, and one that sometimes makes an operation unnecessary. With the pressure under control, the aorta often heals itself, and the patient reports dramatic relief of pain as soon as the pressure is lowered.

# 16

# *Insurance and Other Economic Matters*

Let's face it! It costs money to be sick! If you have been in the hospital recently you know the average room costs a hundred dollars a day, not counting any of the extras.

Remember what we've said before: High blood pressure is the commonest cause of strokes, heart failure, and kidney failure—all of which complications require long hospitalization and, even more important, can be prevented by taking pills and staying under medical care for the rest of your life.

Remember, also, that the milder your disease, the easier it is to treat, and the simpler the treatment, the cheaper the cost.

### The cost

The majority of patients that I see in private practice or in the clinic have mild or moderately severe blood pressure disease, and the majority of these are well-treated with a thiazide diuretic which is usually taken once a day. When the drug is prescribed in large amounts and by its generic (chemical) name, it costs the patient less than two dollars a month. Many doctors, using the same type of therapy, prescribe short-acting drugs which must be given several times a day and, if prescribed by trade name, can cost anywhere from $12.00 to $18.00 a month.

Three brands of the drug reserpine, for example, in one report were found to range from $9.12 to $39.50 per thousand tablets when purchased by brand name, in contrast to the generic price of $1.35 per thousand.

Since there is often a $2.00 charge by pharmacists for every prescription filled, it can save you money to buy a large quantity of pills at one time rather than buying small amounts often.

### High blood pressure drugs and their prices

The following are typical retail prices of high blood pressure drugs in cost per one hundred tablets. The relative costs would be higher if purchased in smaller amounts, and would be lower if purchased in larger amounts.

HydroDiuril, 25 mg., $5.75; 50 mg., $9.75.
Esidrix, 25 mg., $5.75; 50 mg., $8.75.
Naturetin, 5 mg., $7.45; with protein, $8.65.
Naqua, 2 mg., $5.75; 4 mg., $8.75.
Hygroton, 50 mg., $9.75; 100 mg., $11.75.
Lasix, 40 mg., $9.75.
Edecrin, 50 mg., $8.75.
Aldactone, $14.75.
Aldactazide, $14.75.
Dyrenium, 100 mg., $8.75.
Dyazide, $9.75.
Apresoline, 10 mg., $4.25; 25 mg., $5.75; 50 mg., $8.75.
Serpasil, 0.1 mg., $3.95; 0.25 mg., $6.75.
Aldomet, 25 mg., $8.75.
Ismelin, $14.95.
Inderal, 10 mg., $5.75; 40 mg., $8.75.

Even if it costs more than ten dollars a month to bring your high blood pressure under control, all things considered, it is a small price to pay for escaping the risk of a life-shortening or crippling disease.

If you are a businessman used to looking at things from the cost-benefit aspect, then the cost of pills for the rest of your life would certainly seem to be worth the attainment of other values, such as living longer, enjoying one's self, earning a living, having a good family life, being productive, and engaging freely in physical activity.

There are some health insurance plans and systems that pay for most if not all the cost of such drugs.

The average cost of a visit to a physician's office for a high blood pressure check-up and treatment is between $5.00 and $14.00. The cost can often be reduced when a physician uses a nurse or other assistant to see patients for routine pressure readings or when at-home readings are taken and mailed in to the doctor's office.

### What about the costs of tests?

As we discussed earlier, a huge battery of tests is not considered routinely necessary before starting high blood pressure treatment. The recommended tests usually cost about $20.00.

### Does health insurance cover diagnostic costs?

Routine screening for hypertension is not covered by Medicare, Medicaid, or private health insurance companies (except for the periodic screening of children up to age twenty-one allowed by Medicaid). For the past two years, children of families on welfare have been eligible for periodic health screening up to age twenty-one; that program has recently agreed to include blood pressure determinations in the tests to be administered to these young people.

Adults are not covered for screening if they are without symptoms.

But once the diagnosis of hypertension has been made, if you need hospitalization to explore the cause or to assess target organ damage, Medicare, Medicaid, and most private insurance companies will cover that.


### Does health insurance cover drug costs and office visits?

When Medicaid patients are discharged from the hospital, they may or may not be covered for drug costs according to their state's rulings. Most states do allow payment for prescription drugs, but require use of the generic forms at minimal cost.

Usually Medicare patients are not covered for outpatient drugs. But Medicare coverage (Part B) will cover home and office physician visits for "usual and customary" fees.

Task Force IV of the National High Blood Pressure Education Program recommends that states broaden their Medicaid benefits to include reimbursement for services rendered to hypertensive patients by nurses and other paramedical personnel, under the supervision of the physician and employed by him.

They also recommend that all states which do not now do so should change their rules to permit Medicaid coverage of out-patient drugs, and that Medicare should be amended to permit coverage of outpatient anti-hypertensive drugs.

About twenty-five to thirty million people are covered for outpatient drug costs through industrial and other group health contracts with Blue Cross/Blue Shield. Under some company plans, an employee can take a prescription to the pharmacy and be charged $2.00 (or less depending on the contract), regardless of the prescription, and Blue Shield will pay the balance to the pharmacist. Under other contracts, such as for federal employees, Blue Shield will pay for 80 percent of drug costs over $100.00 or $150.00.

When it comes to plans available to the individual, different health insurance plans have differing coverage for office visits, tests, and other out-of-hospital procedures, depending on the options selected and the premiums paid.

## *A pilot study on a new program*

If the asymptomatic patient (and most patients with high blood pressure have no symptoms) is to remain under care and keep taking therapy, he must be motivated, and the only way to motivate him is to establish a meaningful doctor-to-patient relationship. The average physician does not have the time or the interest to develop such a relationship. The nurse or paramedic does. The application of these techniques in a private-practice setting needs to be evaluated. We have, therefore, begun a pilot project in which nurses, specially trained in the treatment of hypertension, have been placed in the office of a general practitioner and in the office of a group of internists. They take the blood pressure of every patient who comes into the doctor's office, and either take over the care of the hypertensive patients entirely from beginning to end or, subject to the discretion of the physician, take over the patient's care when his blood pressure has become normal. The patient then is followed in this way for the rest of his life. Of great importance is the fact that in this pilot demonstration, the Blue Shield organization will pay the patient's bill, just as if the doctor were following the patient.

Hopefully, this project will demonstrate:

1. The large number of undiscovered hypertensive patients in the doctor's office.

2. That the long-term care of most hypertensive patients

is more efficiently handled by a specially trained nurse than by a physician; there will be better blood pressure control, and more patients will keep appointments.

3. As a result, the physician will be given more time to treat the acutely ill patient and the income of his office will be increased.

4. Because of Blue Shield involvement, the practice of preventive medicine will become a definite possibility, that is, asymptomatic patients will be encouraged to come to the physician's office in order to stay well.

## How about getting health insurance?

Most prepaid plans will accept hypertensives without question and at the usual rates, if they join as members of a group. When they apply as individuals and are found to be hypertensive, they occasionally may be refused membership, or charged a higher rate, or asked to sign a waiver exempting the plan from having to pay for any treatment related to that pre-existing condition. If hypertension develops after they are enrolled, they will usually be covered for full diagnostic work-up and in-hospital medication, but not always for outpatient drugs.

Sometimes a special rider is attached to a policy. The person with high blood pressure will be insured, but any episodes of illness or hospitalization attributable to the high pressure are excluded from coverage; expenses incident to their treatment will not be met by the insurer. Due to the complex nature of hypertension, no hard and fast set of rules exists for determining precisely which episodes of illness will be excluded from coverage, so health insurance claims are usually handled on a case-by-case basis, with determinations based on the unique circumstances of each.

One of the best bets if you have high blood pressure is to affiliate with a prepaid medical plan, a group health clinic, or a health maintenance organization. They place their emphasis on preventive medicine, and since it can readily be demonstrated that it is economically advantageous to get hypertensive patients under effective control, these organizations can generally be counted on to screen, verify, diagnose, treat, and follow up all hypertensives detected among their enrollees.

## *Your job*

According to national surveys, people with high blood pressure do not appear to have any significant repercussions on a job because of their high pressure. Only 5 percent of hypertensives report having quit a job because of their high blood pressure. And less than one half of 1 percent said they had ever been fired from a job or refused a promotion because of their high blood pressure.

## *If a checkup shows I have high blood pressure, will my boss be told?*

A boss would not be told by an outside screening program. If you are checked in a company program or by a company doctor, it would depend on what the arrangement was between management and the doctor.

High blood pressure should *not* affect your job. There should be no discrimination against employees who have high blood pressure that is under control.

Unfortunately, occasional employers may use the fact of high blood pressure, or other health conditions, as a basis for refusing to hire or promote someone.

Says Leo Perlis, director of the Department of Community Services of the AFL–CIO: "A great many employees are fearful of losing their jobs should they be discovered to have blood disease or high blood pressure. Job guarantees must be assured and secure. Health insurance coverage must be sustained, and workmen's compensation must not be used by employers to inhibit their employees from seeking information about the state of their health, or from seeking medical assistance when the state of their health requires it."

Dr. Leon Warshaw, chief medical director of the Equitable Life Assurance Society, says that in "most companies—certainly in most large and enlightened companies—there is no discrimination against employees."

And he adds, "In companies with well-established occupational health programs there is indeed an active search for such individuals, and a strong effort made to educate them as to the advisability of treatment."

### High blood pressure and the armed services

Military regulations covering induction physicals require that anyone under age forty whose blood pressure is greater than 140/90 be rejected for military service.

In the past, the military services have had a policy of informing anyone rejected because of elevated blood pressure that he has an abnormal finding, urging him to see his doctor or to go to a clinic. Unfortunately, according to the National High Blood Pressure Education Program, funds to support this minimal service are no longer available.

Hypertension that develops after a man is in the service is not considered a reason for early retirement unless the hypertension does not respond to treatment or is seriously elevated, or unless evidence of target organ damage begins to appear. However, a member of the military will not be sent overseas unless his blood pressure is under good medical control.

The air force standards for flying are a blood pressure reading of less than 140/90 up to the age of thirty-five. Between age thirty-five and forty-five, a reading under

150/90 is necessary. Over age forty-five, less than 154/94 is acceptable.

All military hospitals and outpatient clinics give treatment for hypertension to servicemen and their dependents. Many Veterans Administration hospitals have programs for screening and treating.

## *Life insurance*

Life insurance company executives say high blood pressure is the most prevalent and the most important risk factor producing increased mortality among insurance applicants.

Dr. John Stokes III, executive secretary of the National High Blood Pressure Education Program, headed a study of forty-three life insurance companies and found that most companies will accept persons with high blood pressure. But the cost of premiums is higher for them because of the added risk.

For example, a forty-five-year-old man applying for an ordinary $10,000 whole life policy with no impairments would pay an average premium of about $320.00 per year. If he had a blood pressure reading of 160/100, he would pay an increase of $19.00 per thousand, or a premium of $510.00 per year. With a systolic pressure over 180 or a diastolic over 110 he would pay a $650.00 premium per year!

The size of the extra charge, he found, depends upon the severity of the applicant's condition, his family history, and the presence or absence of related conditions.

It was found that of *all* increased premiums, 40 percent are because of high blood pressure!

Most life insurance companies start charging extra premiums at 140/90 or higher.

One of the interesting sidelights was the finding that many blood pressure levels which are indicative of increased mortality to the insurance industry are not considered serious by most physicians, Dr. Stokes reported. "All the responding medical directors who expressed opinions on this subject felt that many physicians attach too little significance to slightly elevated blood pressure," he said. "However, many felt that a change for the better was occurring in this area as a result of studies establishing the dramatic role of prompt drug treatment in reducing fatalities and morbid incidents among borderline hypertensives."

### If I bring my pressure down, do I save money?

All the responding firms said they reduce premiums if the person presents evidence of an improvement in his condition. However, the amount of pressure reduction and the conditions of treatment under which it may be granted vary within the industry.

Insurance companies usually do not initiate the reviews necessary to lower premiums, but must be requested to do so by the patient, or sometimes the doctor or the insurance agent. There usually is a waiting period of one to two years for re-rating.

Most companies will reduce your premium if your pressure comes down to, say, 135/85 and you keep it there for two years or more. Company requirements vary. You get a rebate if nothing else in your health picture has changed, like gaining lots of weight.

Rating reductions usually come in steps, with a partial reduction given for a person under treatment for six months to two years, a larger reduction given to those who have been treated for more than two years, and so on. Many companies will return to standard ratings if you can keep the pressures down.

You can save money as well as your life by getting and keeping high blood pressure under control!

The saving is 10 to 50 percent, depending on whether you

had straight or term insurance in a life policy. One company estimates a person in his thirties could save $80.00 a year on a $10,000 policy by bringing down previously high pressure. Some companies offer even greater savings. Equitable Life Insurance Company, for example, gives a rating reduction of up to 50 percent with a reading of 139/88 or less. The savings are often more than enough to pay for the pills you have to take.

It should be noted that re-ratings can operate only to the insured individual's benefit. If his blood pressure is demonstrably lower and he has developed no new impairment when he applies for a new rating, his previous rating and thus his premium cost will usually be lowered; if his blood pressure is higher, however, his rating remains the same. Thus it is always to the hypertensive person's advantage to request a re-rating at whatever interval is specified by his insurer.

### *Will my insurance rate rise if I get high blood pressure after my policy was issued?*

No. It stays at the rate it was originally.

# 17

# Research and the Future

It was more than 2,600 years before Christ that a Chinese medical book, a tablet, advised its readers: "When the pulse is stonelike but also like the beating of a hammer, a disease will make its appearance. . . . When the pulse is tense and hard, and full like a cord, there are dropsical swellings." The Chinese treated "hard pulse" with bloodletting and acupuncture, and advised against too much salt.

Egyptian writings, too, spoke of hard pulse, and reports of the Jews, Arabs, Greeks, and Romans spoke of using leeches for bloodletting to treat it. North American and South American Indians bored holes in the skulls of patients.

But it was the year 1711 before blood pressure was actually measured even in a crude way. Stephen Hales, an English clergyman, measured the blood pressure in dogs and horses, using a brass pipe and a glass tube, and was the first to see the rising and falling of the blood pressure with the heartbeat.

He describes opening a mare's left neck artery: "I inserted into it a brass pipe whose bore was one-sixth of an inch in diameter; and to that, by means of another brass pipe which was fitly adapted to it, I fixed a glass tube of nearly the same diameter, which was nine feet in length." He released the ligature around the artery and saw blood rise more than eight feet in the tube. "When it was at its full height," he wrote, "it would rise and fall, at and after each pulse, two, three or four inches."

In 1828, a French medical student, Jean Poiseuille, invented a way to measure blood pressure without making an incision in an artery, and using mercury. Another Frenchman, Julius Hérrison, first observed blood pulsations in man. His instrument consisted of a hollow metal half-ball with a membrane head, with the ball connected to a tube partly filled with mercury. The membrane of the half-ball was placed over the artery in the wrist, and the beat of the pulse would make the mercury bound up and down. Hérrison wrote: "I frequently examine the pulse, and whenever I see that it exceeds the degree of impulse necessary to the equilibrium, I order leeches to be applied, or a certain quantity of blood drawn. I have noticed that loss of blood suffices to bring the pulse back to its normal state. . . ."

That's the treatment there was for high blood pressure: blood-letting, leeches, acupuncture. Even within the last fifty years reported treatments include dilute hydrochloric acid, garlic, cucumber seeds, mistletoe, extract of watermelon, stimulation from an electric current, and bathing in radium water.

Drugs were tried. Some were derived from tobacco cured in fruit. Some were sedatives, so strong that the patient walked around in a constant semi-stupor, alive but half asleep. None did much good.

Surgery was successful in some patients. Some surgeons tried removing kidney tissue, some sectioned nerves coming from the carotid sinus, or other nerves. The most effective surgical treatment—but also the most drastic—was controlling severe forms of hypertension by cutting the main trunk of sympathetic nerve fibers that carried impulses to the blood vessels. The procedure, called sympathectomy, stopped the stimulation of the blood vessels and so usually controlled the hypertension, but it also produced many inconvenient side effects such as dizziness on standing, pain for six to twelve months after surgery, and frequent incidence of sexual impairment.

Today, the procedure is no longer necessary because of the modern high blood pressure drugs that we now have.

But it was the 1960s before we really knew drugs made a difference.

Dr. Irvine Page, director emeritus of research at Cleveland Clinic, describes pre-drug times in an interview in Medical Tribune's *Hypertension Bulletin.* "The more I studied hypertension—beginning around 1928 or 1929—the more it seemed to me that this was a new class of diseases," he said. "We always hoped we'd find a bacteria, a virus, or something that would, you know, be a single cause for it. And this never worked. All we kept getting was more and more substances, more and more things that seemed to regulate blood pressure.

"When I proposed the mosaic theory, everybody said, 'Well it's an awfully nice theory and very nice of you, because you include my work and everybody else's, but it doesn't mean anything.'

"Many people did not believe that you should lower blood pressure—a very convenient theory, because we didn't know how to lower it. When I was in medical school, for instance, we had a comfortable advantage, for we had never heard of a heart attack. Myocardial infarction did not even exist.

"It was believed in those days that if you lowered pressure this would produce inadequate perfusion of the tissues because of the thickening of the blood vessels, and therefore treatment would definitely be damaging. So, that settled the problem of treatment—you did not have to treat.

"Fortunately, treatment has outstripped our understanding of the thing, so that we now have available many treatments that we are not really entitled to."

## *Progress is made*

Things finally started falling into place. In 1918, Dr. James B. Herrick of Chicago, the man who just a few years earlier had first described sickle cell anemia, made the first diagnosis of heart attack. Up until then no correlation had been made between chest pain, sudden death, and the heart. Chest pain, doctors thought, was caused by indigestion.

The well-known Dr. William Osler suggested a link between chest pain and blood pressure. Dr. S. A. Levine, an American cardiologist, reported that 60 percent of his heart attack patients had high blood pressure and that it was probably the most common cause of heart attacks.

In 1948, investigators reported they found more than four times more heart attack deaths in soldiers with high blood pressure than in those with normal pressures.

Then came the insurance study showing that life expectancy was significantly lower in people who had high blood pressure, and the life-shortening effect could even be seen in people who had only mildly elevated pressures.

Just after World War II, it was accidentally discovered that a malaria drug called pentaquine not only was effective against malaria, but also lowered blood pressure in the men it was tested on. It was tried on a physician who had desperately high pressure and was rapidly approaching death. He had a diastolic (lower) pressure of 160! With the pentaquine his pressure fell to 100, his severe headaches disappeared, and signs of heart failure began to ease away. It was the first time that high blood pressure had been successfully treated with a drug.

Now investigators started looking for other drugs in earnest.

Veratrum, the medicinal herb used by American Indians, was tried. Injected into veins of high blood pressure patients, it did lower pressure, and dramatically cleared many symptoms, but there were often severe reactions to the drug with violent nausea, sweating, and collapse.

In really severe cases, doctors sometimes tried combined therapy: the veratrum, plus the sympathectomy operation, plus the then-in-vogue low-salt rice diet.

The drug hexamethonium was found by British investigators to be effective in lowering pressure, but it had to be injected several times a day, and so was used in only the most severe cases.

It was in the late 1950s that thiazides were discovered. A derivative of the old infection-fighting sulfa drugs, they were found to increase the kidney's excretion of sodium and water, and so lowered blood pressure. And now today, just a few years after the serious search for effective high blood pressure drugs began, the thiazides are our mainstay of treatment and, together with other new drugs, are saving hundreds of thousands of lives.

### Research today

In our progress against high blood pressure, the biggest step has been the new drugs.

Twenty years ago, there was almost nothing that could be done for high blood pressure. Ten years ago we had drugs, but doctors weren't convinced they really did any good in preventing stroke or heart damage. Now we have the drugs and we have the data that show that they truly do work in preventing disability and early death.

But we still have a long way to go. The disease still claims hundreds of thousands of lives.

Even though we have good treatment available, people are not getting it.

We still don't know the cause of most high blood pressure. And because we don't know the cause, or causes, we have no effective way to prevent it from developing.

To help solve some of these problems, hundreds of

research projects are being carried out in hospitals and medical schools throughout the world. Projects that range from searching for the causes of high blood pressure to exploring for better ways to convince people to get their blood pressure checked and to follow directions to keep pressure under control.

### *Ferreting out the still mysterious causes*

Much of research is basic—studying the function of the kidneys and the action of hormones and the anatomy of blood vessels—trying to learn just what the causes and mechanisms of high blood pressure are. What really happens in the body as hormones, and chemicals, and various influences work on each other? The interrelationships are so complex that computer systems have been set up to study them.

Heredity is being studied. So is diet, salt, chemicals in the water, and other environmental factors. So are psychological factors, infectious agents and many other possibilities. The liver is being implicated as a factor, particularly regarding its ability to metabolize certain hormones.

### *Better diagnosis*

The standard way of measuring the blood pressure with the sphygmomanometer is a good one, but researchers are trying to find an even better one, one that would be especially quick and accurate for mass screening and for home measurements. Several new ones are now being put on the market and are being evaluated. New instruments are also being developed for continuous automatic recording of pressure throughout the day.

Laboratory tests are being perfected for better diagnosis of the more rare forms of high blood pressure, to find more and more cases with the kinds of high pressure that can be permanently cured.

Researchers at Duke University are working on a test to measure how much of a certain enzyme is released in a person's blood by nerve endings. The level found may make it possible to pick out people who are likely to develop high blood pressure even before they begin to show signs. The test may also be valuable in establishing diagnosis when pressures change so much from measurement to measurement that doctors don't know whether to diagnose hypertension or not.

To try to make diagnosis more precise than it is now, Dr. John Laragh, of Columbia-Presbyterian Medical Center in New York, performs what he calls "hormone profiling" of patients to try to determine what drug might be most effective for their hypertension. Treatment can often be tailored so that an effective drug can be chosen without as many trials, says Dr. Laragh.

He and associates measure the amount of two hormones —the kidney hormone, renin, which raises blood pressure, and an adrenal gland hormone, aldosterone, which causes salt and water to be retained in the body.

The different hormones may be involved in producing high blood pressure in different patients.

"If you know the hormone levels, you can pick the right drug," Laragh says. "We believe we now can spot patients with biochemical defects, and subdivide them into groups for the best specific treatment."

It is hoped that research in the renin-aldosterone field may give insight into the basic mechanisms of high blood pressure—what really causes it.

At Michael Reese Hospital and Medical Center in Chicago, Dr. Fredric L. Coe is developing a computer to diagnose and prescribe treatment for patients with high blood pressure. In the Michael Reese Clinic, a physician gives each patient a physical examination, orders lab tests, and measures the blood pressure. These data are fed into the computer, which has been intricately programmed with information on high blood pressure. Within a few minutes, a printout of recommendations appears. The recommendations may be simple, telling a new patient to come back for more blood pressure readings, or may designate specific changes in drugs and dosage. The recommendations go to the patient's doctor, who can okay them or rewrite them.

## *Even better drugs*

We have some excellent drugs now, but some of them do have side effects, so drug companies are all working feverishly to come up with more efficient drugs with smaller dosages needed and fewer side effects.

Some of these are already undergoing clinical trials.

For example, a new drug, minoxidil—which can be taken in pill form once a day—has been very effective in patients with severe forms of high blood pressure. Similar to more potent drugs, it causes retention of fluid (which can be treated by giving a diuretic). Its only limiting feature (particularly in women) is the stimulation of hair growth.

Several other very potent blood pressure lowering drugs already available in Europe are currently being evaluated in this country in the Veteran Administration hospitals.

The main active ingredient in marijuana is being studied for blood pressure lowering effects at McGill University in Montreal. It is proving very effective in animal studies.

The new promising compounds called prostaglandins (named because they were believed to be related to the prostate gland) are being looked at with tremendous interest also. They not only have been found to lower blood pressure, but also have been found to improve kidney function. First found in semen, now in some forms made synthetically, they may be an important high blood pressure medicine of the future.

Other drugs are on the drawing boards or are being tested in animals.

## Mind over matter

We've already told you the exciting things going on in the use of biofeedback and other visceral training to control blood pressure.

Now, research is being done with electrosleep therapy, the technique of sleeping while being stimulated with low frequency electric impulses. In Bulgaria, Prof. Dr. V. Sirakiva reports that electrosleep sessions lowered blood pressure as well as serum cholesterol levels; and in Moscow, using electrosleep, Prof. Dr. L. A. Studnizyna found improvement in 83 percent of 135 patients with high blood pressure.

Yoga and other relaxation exercises are being studied scientifically, also. In England, Dr. C. H. Patel used these techniques along with biofeedback successfully to lower high blood pressure in a number of patients. In a few patients, control was so good that they were able to stop taking medication for their high pressure.

Since the study was just completed we do not know how long the effects will last, or how long the patients will keep up their relaxation exercises, but Dr. Patel calls yoga, biofeedback, and other relaxation techniques, "a useful new approach" to treatment of high blood pressure.

## Other research on treatment

New or renewed looks are being taken in other directions also. At Hahnemann Medical College in Philadelphia, for example, researchers are implanting an electronic device right into the neck muscle that puts out a current to stimulate the nerves in the carotid sinus, the center that is one of the controllers of the body's blood pressure. The stimulator is run by a battery-pack worn outside the body. So far the device is being used on patients who don't respond to drug therapy, and is proving effective in bringing high pressures down to near normal.

Other doctors are looking at the ratio of calcium to sodium in the body, wondering whether that is a key to high blood pressure in addition to salt intake, and whether decreasing calcium intake might lower pressure.

And a fresh look is being taken at other risk factors, too, both in relation to high blood pressure and in relation to heart attacks and stroke. In a group of more than a dozen medical centers across the United States, evaluation programs are being carried out with more than ten thousand people to see on a mass scale what a really concerted effort attacking all of the risk factors—like smoking and obesity—can do toward lowering the shocking rate of heart attack and stroke in our population.

### Completing the statistical picture

Astonishingly enough, with high blood pressure so thoroughly researched in some areas, we are missing very basic data in other areas.

For example—women liberationists arise—almost all the data that we have on high blood pressure at this time are on men. We don't really have accurate statistics on women.

Similarly, there are no data on patients who only have an increase in their systolic pressure. Does treating these patients do any good?

Another statistical gap: We don't have data from large numbers of people on the benefits of treatment on mild and borderline cases of high blood pressure, that is, diastolic pressure of 90 to 104. We have statistics from small studies, but not as we do for severe and moderate hypertension. This is being corrected however by a study now underway by the

U.S. Public Health Service on mild hypertension. And the study is already showing that reducing blood pressure does help prevent complications even when blood pressure is only slightly elevated. The incidence of stroke, eye damage, heart enlargement, and more severe hypertension are all being significantly reduced.

The same sort of gap in statistics occurs with the question of whether reducing high blood pressure reduces heart attacks. We know it makes a huge life-saving difference in preventing strokes, heart failure, and kidney breakdown, but the prevention programs have not given us the same clear-cut statistics on heart attacks. A number of studies have suggested that controlling high blood pressure does decrease the incidence of heart attacks, and others have shown that lowering the blood pressure in patients with heart disease lowers the severity and frequency of angina pain; (many in fact have been able to stop taking their angina medicine when they got their blood pressure down to normal). But we don't have studies on *large numbers* of people, or studies where high blood pressure therapy was begun in the early stages.

So what is needed at this time is a study of treatment of mild hypertension in men and women *at early ages*, and with the study lasting some ten years, so that the differences in heart attack rates have time to show up. Such a study is now starting, under the direction of Dr. H. Mitchell Perry, chief of medical services at the Veterans Administration Hospital in St. Louis. The project will be carried out in twenty medical centers with some eight thousand people. We're expecting it to show a cut in heart attack rate of at least 50 percent.

### Reaching the people

Research is not just what goes on in a laboratory or in a hospital, it can also involve health delivery, the best ways to reach and treat the public. All the new research and all the great treatments in the world aren't going to help the people who have high blood pressure unless we find them and motivate them to stay on that treatment.

Through the gray bleakness of most clinic programs there are several excellent programs that light the way for what could be. They illustrate the possibilities of simpler history taking, better communication techniques, and the use of non-physician personnel.

One of these is the AMOS program at DeWitt Army Hospital in Ft. Belvoir, Virginia. AMOS stands for *Automated Military Outpatient System*. Begun in 1969, its goal was to computerize the outpatient health care of the army hospital to make it more efficient. Before that, patients often waited as long as three hours to see a physician. A survey showed that thirty common complaints accounted for 80 percent of the walk-in problems. A set of rules for treating each clinical problem was designed by physicians, and paraprofessionals were trained to use them in processing patients. They advise about half the patients themselves and refer another half to physicians.

In the acute minor illness clinic, four to six paramedics perform most of the diagnosis and treatment on minor illnesses under the supervision of a doctor, seeing between them 126 patients on an average day. Patients seldom wait more than thirty minutes.

In the chronic care program, where hypertension is handled, a physician is responsible for evaluation of the problem and prescription of treatment, and a nurse is responsible for most of the patient education and support. Both doctor and nurse are responsible for follow-up of patients.

At almost the same time AMOS was set up, the Atlanta Community High Blood Pressure Program also began. Its goal—to see if widespread community methods could improve the control of hypertension. The area selected was a low-income, predominately black area in central Atlanta.

Blood pressure technicians—neighborhood women with no previous medical experience—were trained to do interviews and measure blood pressures.

Of six thousand people screened initially, about 30 percent were found to be hypertensive and were referred to their physicians for care. Approximately three to nine months later they were contacted again for rescreening and to see if they had sought treatment and continued it.

Later treatment facilities were set up in the neighborhood and staffed with nurses, a social worker, a blood pressure technician, and two part-time physicians. Nurses were responsible for the follow-up of the hypertensives, making recommendations for treatment, which were reviewed by the doctor.

The Harlem Hospital Hypertension and Stroke Control Project also uses community health workers. Health workers are recruited in Harlem and given six months training in preventive medicine, high blood pressure, and problems such as drug and alcohol abuse. Workers move freely and with little fear in Harlem, making home visits where others would not go.

The Boston Ambulatory Care Project uses high school graduates without previous medical experience as health assistants to carry out many functions.

And we have already told you of the success in our D.C. General Clinic in Washington, using paramedical personnel and other techniques to decrease dropout rates. Since our reorganization, 92 percent of our patients have stayed with us instead of the huge dropout we had before.

# 18

# Where Do We Go from Here?

Why has high blood pressure been so ignored except for a few programs?

Part of the problem has been with the nature of the disease itself. Despite the fact that it is a serious disease, people who have it don't necessarily feel bad, so they don't go to the doctor, and when they do find out that their pressure is high, they often don't follow treatment advice.

Part of the problem is with the nature of our society. We tend to give more money and attention to the diseases that are dramatic than we do to the ones that are less so, even though the latter diseases may kill and cripple more people in the long run. We also tend to not do the things that we know we should, even when we know that they are good for us and will make us feel better or live longer.

Part of the blame rests with physicians who, like their patients, have failed to take the problem of high blood pressure seriously, who have been slow to take up the new knowledge about the life-saving value of lowering blood pressure, who have remained unconvinced that the benefits of treatment are worth the expense and inconvenience.

And part of the blame lies with the medical societies and

medical communicators who have not gotten the message about the seriousness of high blood pressure to either the public or to enough physicians.

But now much of that is changing.

Government programs are being set up. Screening is being done from city to city. The message about high blood pressure is being broadcast across the world in brochures, in newspapers and magazines, on radio and on television. Information is being sent to all physicians and to all medical societies on the recommended treatments for high pressure. State and community programs are mushrooming. Pharmaceutical houses are sponsoring education packets and programs. Medical journals are featuring editorials and articles on the values and needs for treatment.

The truth is finally getting out. We're feeling a new optimism, and we're finally seeing a little action.

## The National High Blood Pressure Education Program

The meeting of medical leaders described at the very beginning of this book was responsible for some of that action. From that group and others four government task forces were formed to investigate and make recommendations about:

1. screening, referral, and treatment
2. educating professionals about high blood pressure
3. educating the public
4. assessing the ability of the health care system to handle the increased diagnostic and treatment load

A committee was formed—the National High Blood Pressure Education Committee—that was made up of representatives of the National Heart and Lung Institute, the Veterans Administration, the American Heart Association, the American Medical Association, the National Medical Association, and other medical organizations and societies, both public and private.

Funded by only $2 million dollars from the federal government, the committee is nevertheless spearheading a campaign across the country that is involving people in all social and economic classes and from every walk of life: professional and volunteer groups, pharmaceutical companies, industry and labor, local communities, and individual physicians and laymen. It even crosses national boundaries, with cooperative projects beginning with the World Health Organization and private foundations of several countries. Pilot programs for controlling high blood pressure have already been launched in ten countries by WHO.

Surveys were done of current attitudes and opinions on high blood pressure held by the public, and a survey is also being done on the attitudes of doctors. Workshops are being held for members of the medical profession and community leaders, so that education, screening, and treatment programs can be set up by communities themselves on a local level. Experts from around the world have worked for months preparing instructions on recommended treatments, so that physicians would have standard guidelines to follow with their patients. Books, cassettes, and films have been prepared with information for the public and for physicians.

Insurance companies have been surveyed to learn how high blood pressure affects a person's life and health insurance rates.

Television spots and full-length documentaries have been prepared; newspaper and magazine articles have been written; radio talks given. Brochures have been written and distributed both by the national government, by private agencies such as the American Heart Association, and by pharmaceutical companies.

The National Red Cross has agreed to screen all blood donors for high blood pressure. The American Medical Association has officially recommended to their entire membership that every doctor, no matter whether a general practitioner or a specialist, routinely take and at least annually repeat blood pressure measurements on all patients. They have set up a special committee on hypertension to make further recommendations.

The American Heart Association has named high blood pressure its major area of emphasis in their current fight against heart disease.

The American College of Cardiology is initiating special symposiums for physicians on high blood pressure.

Screening programs have been carried out in hundreds of local communities, reaching hundreds of thousands of people. In one program, even school children are being taught to take blood pressure so that in the sixth grade they are aware of what high blood pressure is and what it means. And they go home and take their parents' pressures and bring back the reports!

## The High Blood Pressure Information Center

A center has been established at the National Institute of Health for collection and dissemination of public and professional information about high blood pressure as a part of the national blood pressure program.

There brochures, produced by the government, are available, as well as films, cassettes, TV documentaries, and exhibits. And there are lists of all materials and supplies on high blood pressure that are produced by other groups, so the center is acting as a complete national clearinghouse of information and material.

The center also has charts for schools, displays, and exhibits for conventions and meetings, and speakers available for large or small groups. They have material for workshops for groups who wish to set up local screening, educational, or treatment programs. And they have consultation services with experts available to work with groups who want to set up community action programs, whether they are grade school students or university hospital personnel. Physicians also can use the center for answers to questions, referrals, reprints of journal articles, guidelines from the task forces, and other aids.

The Information Center address is:

National High Blood Pressure Information Center
120/80 National Institute of Health
Bethesda, Maryland   20014

## *The American Heart Association*

The national and local chapters of the American Heart Association also have a great deal of material on high blood pressure. For television stations there are TV spots and documentaries, for meetings and schools there are films, displays and brochures, for physicians there are pamphlets on office evaluation of high blood pressure, drug treatment of high pressure, and materials that can be given to patients.

For further information on specific materials available, contact your local heart association, or write to:

American Heart Association
   Attention: Material Development Dept.
44 East 23rd Street
New York, NY   10010

## *Citizens for Treatment of High Blood Pressure, Inc.*

This non-profit organization was begun early in 1973 to marshal private and voluntary resources for the fight on high blood pressure.

Supported and guided by a group of distinguished citizens deeply concerned with public health, the committee is undertaking educational projects in collaboration with existing private, voluntary, and public organizations. They stand by to implement and expand programs already underway, and to stimulate new programs and ideas.

Their current emphasis has been to focus increased attention on untreated high blood pressure and its consequences, by working with national media, local officials, members of Congress, industry, organized labor, and professional health organizations.

One of the founders of the group, Mary Lasker—president of the Albert and Mary Lasker Foundation and a person who has crusaded for many health causes—was also instrumental in getting Elliot Richardson, then Secretary of Health, Education and Welfare, to call the first meeting and to launch the current national high blood pressure program.

## The remaining needs

All of these programs have produced some major steps toward improving care in people with high blood pressure, in saving lives.

There is still much to be done.

High blood pressure is still the leading reason for patient visits to most private practitioners. The average practitioner sees twenty to forty patients a week with high blood pressure. And this is just the tip of the iceberg, because at least twice as many people should be coming in.

There are still millions of people who don't know they have the disease or who are not getting proper treatment.

There are still unnecessary deaths.

## The costs of high blood pressure

We can talk about the economic costs to the United States of cardiovascular disease—medical services, research, lost wages. High blood pressure, since it is the leading risk factor in cardiovascular disease, is a big part of that. The American Heart Association says the cost last year for cardiovascular disease was $19.5 billion. The U.S. Public Health Service estimates $30.5 billion for direct and indirect cardiovascular patient costs! Some of this disease and some of the deaths were due to other factors also; high blood pressure doesn't cause *all* heart and circulatory disease—but high blood pressure certainly accounts for an important part of those financial costs.

We can talk about the cost of expensive long-term care for the disabled elderly, money that could be saved, as well as misery prevented.

We can talk about the loss of productivity. High blood pressure often occurs in young and middle-aged adults, where disability and premature death is so tragic and the costs so great.

The disease is still responsible for an estimated 450 million days of restricted activity, 160 million days of disability in bed, and 6 billions of dollars of lost productivity every year.

The most recent records show that of one year's worker disability allowances, 24 percent were due to diseases of the circulatory system, with arteriosclerotic heart disease at the top of the list. How much of this was due in part to high blood pressure? Certainly a third, perhaps more. Hypertensive heart disease appears among the *top* disability causes for blacks.

Mr. Clarence Randall, president of Inland Steel Company in Chicago, did a study on this. After having a heart attack himself, alone in a hotel room in a foreign country, he became highly sensitized to the cardiovascular disease problem. He went back to his plant and asked how many disabilities and deaths were occurring from coronaries and how many were resulting from injuries. The ratio was about 60 to 1, with cardiovascular disease deaths overwhelmingly more common than those from injuries. He then found that even though the plant had a great safety program to prevent such injuries, there was no program to prevent cardiovascular disabilities. A totally irrational situation both from a human and monetary cost viewpoint that is repeated in company after company throughout the nation.

What all this adds up to is that high blood pressure and its complications are the major producers of labor force disability today!

How much of this disability and death could be spared by finding and controlling high blood pressure! Think what an investment in a control program would yield year by year in terms of reduced cost for disability and death, hospitalization and absenteeism. One expert estimates: $35 *billion!*

Like other preventive medicine undertakings to control mass disease, controlling high blood pressure in this country would more than pay for itself financially. It should be less expensive to find and control blood pressure on a mass scale than to care for those who become disabled and economically unproductive as a result of the disease.

Just think if we could postpone the onset of cardiovascular disease for only five to ten years in the average person's lifetime—a very reasonable goal—think of the billions of dollars that could be saved.

These are the economic costs. The real costs are in human terms: the incalculable tragedy of impaired lives, unnecessary suffering and death.

### *A recommended program of action*

Many recommendations have been made in the last few years about what should be done about high blood pressure and what should be done to combat the epidemic of heart disease we are now experiencing. In 1970 and 1971 for example, the Inter-Society Commission for Heart Disease Resources, an organization of representatives of twenty-nine leading health organizations, developed guidelines for what was needed. They came out with three reports that outlined problems and recommendations to solve them.

Other groups have made recommendations, also.

Some of these have been carried out. Some have not.

The following are the fifteen action steps that we think are vital to a successful battle against high blood pressure.

• Increase in screening, using available resources: schools, employment physicals, already existing mobile units, hospitals. We need every physician and every clinic and every hospital in existence today to take blood pressure measurements on every patient who walks in their doors.

• Increase and improvement in follow-up procedures. It doesn't do any good to screen people and find who has high blood pressure if you don't get them to the doctor for further evaluation and treatment.

• Increase in the training and use of paramedical personnel. Nurses, ex-medical corpsmen, medical assistants, community volunteers, and even high school students can be easily trained to take blood pressure measurements and counsel patients. Only by using these trained assistants can we provide the necessary time and attention to educating and treating the large number of people who have high blood pressure.

• Use of other allied medical groups. Dentists, pharmacists, nurses and others can all have a vital role in the campaign against high blood pressure, and should be encouraged to develop programs.

• Stepped-up physician education, stressing the seriousness of high blood pressure and the importance of proper early treatment—*before* damage is done. This would include new emphasis in medical school training as well as postgraduate refresher training. Every teaching hospital should have a clinic for training physicians and paramedical personnel in diagnosis and treatment of high blood pressure.

• Clinics need to be reorganized so that patient waiting

time is reduced. Clinics should be run for the convenience of the patients, not the convenience of the staff, so patients will keep appointments, lose less time from work, and keep up with treatments.

• A coordinated public education effort on the dangers of high blood pressure and the benefits of treatment. These educational programs should include information on the need for continuing medication as well as advice on other risk factors for heart attack and stroke, such as smoking and obesity and what should be done to control them. Special attention must be given to reach all racial and ethnic groups.

• School educational programs should be set up to include information on high blood pressure and nutrition and the hazards of smoking, obesity, and high cholesterol diets.

• A redesign of medical insurance to cover the cost of outpatient visits and of drugs prescribed for long term treatment of high blood pressure. Medicare, Medicaid, Blue Cross, and others should be persuaded to extend their policies for such coverage, since preventive care is more economical in the long run than emergency care of crises and complications. And they should allow payment to be made for services provided by medical assistants under the supervision of a doctor.

• State laws should be changed. Legislation authorizing physician assistants and qualified allied health personnel to provide services to patients under physician supervision should be passed in all states which have not already done so.

• Life insurance companies should adjust their premium ratings so that the patient with controlled high blood pressure would be categorized at no greater risk of premature death than the person with normally low pressure.

• The Joint Commission on the Accreditation of Hospitals should require for hospital accreditation that all patients entering any hospital have a blood pressure reading taken with their complete physical examination.

• Food manufacturers should be encouraged to produce Prudent Diet foods and in other ways to help reshape people's dangerous and self-destructive eating habits. Manufacturers of baby food should be forbidden to add salt to baby food.

• Physicians should include education on modifying diet patterns and other risk factors such as cigarette smoking as part of their regular office practice. This can be done through direct counselling, through use of paramedical assistants, or with literature racks. Sale of cigarettes should be banned from all medical facilities.

• Patients should be told their actual blood pressure numbers when their blood pressure readings are taken. They should remember them, or keep records of them, just as they do their weight, blood type and other vital medical information. The more patients know about their own health, the more they can do to keep it in good shape.

This program would mean that millions of people would enjoy many extra and better years of life.

### *Is there anything you can do?*

First, you will help just by knowing the facts. Knowing the facts, you can help spread the word about the real dangers of high blood pressure.

You can help plan high blood pressure programs in your own organization or community, whether it be through school, church, work, fraternal group or local hospital. You know your area and your neighbors and how best they might be reached.

You can work as a volunteer in screening or other high blood pressure programs. Check the National High Blood

Pressure Center or your local chapter of the American Heart Association for ongoing programs in your area.

And above all, have your blood pressure checked. And the blood pressures of every member of your family, including the kids. If someone close to you has high blood pressure, show concern and encourage them to take their medication and follow whatever advice the doctor gives them.

Down with high blood pressure. Down with people who say "It's only your nerves." Down with doctors who say "It's only up a little, let's not worry about it now."

We want you and your family to have the best chance in the world to have the longest and greatest life possible.

# Appendix A: How to Take a Blood Pressure Reading

Taking a blood pressure is fairly simple to do. You will need a blood pressure machine called a sphygmomanometer and a stethoscope. (Some machines have a meter and do not need a stethoscope. These instructions are for those with a stethoscope.)

It is best not to take your own pressure, since bending to get in the right position can change the pressure. Have a friend or someone in your family do it. It is also best to have a nurse or doctor or other knowledgeable person show you how to do it the first time.

*Be quiet.* Arrange for a quiet place to do the measurement. There should be a table and two chairs.

*Bare arm.* The "patient" should bare the arm well above the elbow and sit down comfortably. There should be no conversation while the blood pressure is being taken.

*Put on cuff.* Apply the blood pressure cuff flatly and snugly on the bare arm above the elbow.

*Raise arm.* Raise the "patient's" arm above the shoulder and then rapidly pump up the cuff until the pressure gauge reads 250 mm Hg.

*Lower arm.* Lower the arm to the table, with the elbow extended.

*Apply stethoscope.* (Ear tips face forward.) Place the stethoscope bell flat on the soft flesh in the inside of the crook of the elbow and let the air out of the cuff so that the needle on the pressure gauge (or the level of mercury) falls about 2 mm Hg with each heartbeat.

*Listen for blood sounds—systolic pressure.* As the pressure in the cuff falls you will hear a distinct thudding noise in the stethoscope. The pressure at which this begins is the *systolic blood pressure.*

*Diastolic pressure.* As you continue to let the air out of the cuff, the thudding noises will stop. The pressure at which this stops is the *diastolic blood pressure.* If the noise does not stop you will notice a pressure at which the sound changes markedly, and this can be taken as the diastolic pressure.

# Appendix B: The Ten Most Important Things to Remember About High Blood Pressure

High blood pressure is a serious condition. If untreated, it is the major cause of strokes, heart failure, and kidney failure. It often leads to early death.

These tragic complications can often be prevented if high blood pressure is treated early.

Millions of people have high blood pressure—at least one in every ten people. It can strike children and adults, men and women, people of all races.

Most people who have high blood pressure don't know they have it.

In its early stages there are no symptoms. You can feel well and still be in danger of your life.

It is easy to detect. A blood pressure test is inexpensive, quick, painless.

High blood pressure can be treated. Treatment is simple. A pill or more a day can usually bring your blood pressure down.

You must take your pills every day, even when you feel well. You should call your doctor when you do not feel well.

High blood pressure does not go away. Treatment is

usually lifelong and should never be discontinued unless a physician specifically says to stop.

A person can lead a normal life if he begins treatment early and keeps it up.

# *Appendix C: Medical Identification Card*

If you have high blood pressure, have a copy of this identification card made and place it in your wallet where it can be seen in any emergency.

---

## MEDICAL IDENTIFICATION CARD

I am taking the following medications for high blood pressure:
(indicate drug names and dosages)

_____     _____

_____     _____

Other drugs for other conditions being taken are:
(indicate condition and medicine)

_____     _____

_____     _____

Doctor's name:_____     My name:_____
Telephone Number:_____     Address:_____
                                      Telephone Number:_____

# *Glossary*

ADRENALIN: A secretion of the adrenal glands, located just above the kidneys. Also called epinephrine. Sometimes prepared synthetically. Constricts the small blood vessels, increases the rate of heart beat, and raises blood pressure.

ALDOSTERONE: A hormone secreted by the adrenal cortex that promotes the conservation of salt and water by the kidneys.

ANGINA PECTORIS: Chest pain because the heart muscle receives an insufficient blood supply. Pain sometimes is also referred down the left arm and forearm.

ANGIOTENSIN: A powerful blood vessel constrictor generated from a protein in the blood through the action of renin, an enzyme released from the kidney.

ANTI-HYPERTENSIVE AGENTS: Drugs used to lower blood pressure.

ANXIETY: A feeling of apprehension.

AORTA: The large artery coming from the left ventricle of the heart.

APOPLEXY: Also called apoplectic stroke or stroke. Due to interruption of the blood supply to a part of the brain caused by the obstruction or rupture of an artery, thereby causing brain damage. This may cause loss of consciousness, loss of speech or hearing, and may leave a part of the body temporarily or permanently paralyzed.

ARRHYTHMIA: An irregular rhythm of the heart beat.

ARTERIES: Major vessels carrying blood from the heart.

ARTERIOLES: Small arteries.

ARTERIOSCLEROSIS: Degeneration or hardening of the arteries.

ATHEROSCLEROSIS: Deposits of cholesterol or lipid material in the arteries.

AUTONOMIC NERVOUS SYSTEM: That portion of the nervous system concerned with unconscious or involuntary functions of the body. Divided into parasympathetic and sympathetic nervous systems.

CAPILLARIES: Small blood vessels or channels between arteries and veins.

CARDIOVASCULAR: Referring to the heart and blood vessels.

CARDIAC: Pertaining to the heart. Sometimes refers to a person who has heart disease.

CARDIOVASCULAR-RENAL DISEASE: Disease involving the heart, blood vessels, and kidneys.

CATHETERIZATION: The process of examining the heart by means of introducing a thin tube (catheter) into a vein or artery and passing it into the heart.

CEREBRAL-VASCULAR ACCIDENT: Sometimes called CVA, apoplectic stroke, or simply stroke. Due to an impeded blood supply to some part of the brain, generally caused by a blood clot forming in the vessel (cerebral thrombosis); a rupture of the blood vessel wall (cerebral hemorrhage); a piece of clot or other material from another part of the vascular system which flows to the brain and obstructs a cerebral vessel (cerebral embolism); or pressure on a blood vessel as by a tumor.

CEREBROVASCULAR: Pertaining to the blood vessels in the brain.

CHOLESTEROL: One of the lipid (fat) substances of the body; a key chemical involved in the development of atherosclerosis. Found in animal tissue. In blood tests, the normal level for Americans is considered to be between 180 and 230 milligrams of cholesterol for each 100 cubic centimeters of blood.

COARCTATION OF THE AORTA: A pressing together, or narrowing, of the aorta, which is the main trunk artery which conducts blood from the heart to the body. One of the several types of congenital heart defects. Can cause high blood pressure.

COLLATERAL CIRCULATION: Circulation of the blood through nearby smaller vessels in order to compensate for blockage of a main vessel.

Congestive heart failure: Loss of efficiency of pumping action of the heart resulting in accumulation of fluid in the tissues and a generalized sluggishness in the circulation. The eventual backing-up of fluid in the lungs results in shortness of breath, first on exertion and later at rest.

Constriction: Narrowing of the internal diameter of blood vessels caused either by contraction of the muscular coat or by thickening, thus encroaching on the passageway of the blood vessel.

Coronary arteries: Arteries arising from the aorta, arching down over the top of the heart, supplying blood to the heart muscle.

Coronary atherosclerosis: An irregular thickening of the inner layer of the walls of the arteries which conduct blood to the heart muscle. The internal channel of these arteries becomes narrowed and the blood supply to the heart muscle is reduced. *See Atherosclerosis.*

Coronary occlusion: An obstruction in a branch of a coronary artery which blocks the flow of blood to a part of heart muscle. The part of the heart muscle supplied by this artery then dies because of lack of blood supply.

Coronary thrombosis: The blockage of the coronary artery is referred to as coronary thrombosis (occlusion). The result is death of heart muscle, i.e., myocardial infarction.

Decompensation: Inability of the heart to maintain adequate circulation, usually resulting in a waterlogging of tissues. A person whose heart is failing to maintain normal circulation is said to be "decompensated."

Diastolic: Blood pressure present during relaxation of the heart or that pressure necessary to overcome resistance of the column of blood to flow through the smallest arteries (arterioles).

Digitalis: A cardiac stimulant increasing contractility of heart muscle.

Digitalized: The process of giving the proper amount of digitalis.

Dilation: A stretching or enlargement of the heart or blood vessels beyond the norm.

DIURESIS: Increased excretion of urine.

DIURETIC: A medicine which promotes the excretion of urine. Several types of drugs may be used, such as mercurials or thiazides.

EDEMA: Swelling due to abnormally large amounts of fluid in the tissues of the body.

ELECTROCARDIOGRAM (ECG or EKG): Measurement on graph paper of electrical activity of heart muscle.

EMBOLUS: A blood clot (or other substance such as air, fat, tumor), inside a blood vessel which is carried in the blood stream to a smaller vessel where it becomes an obstruction to circulation.

EPINEPHRINE: One of the secretions of the adrenal glands. Also called adrenalin. Constricts the small blood vessels.

ESSENTIAL HYPERTENSION: Hypertension without a known specific cause (the commonest type).

FIBRILLATION: Uncoordinated contractions of the heart muscle occurring when the individual muscle fibers take up independent irregular contractions.

FUNDUS OF EYE: The inside of the back part of the eye seen by looking through the pupil with a special light (ophthalmoscope). Examining the fundus of the eye is used as a means of assessing changes in the blood vessels. Also called *eyeground*.

HEART BLOCK: Interference with the conduction of the electrical impulses of the heart which can be either partial or complete. This can result in dissociation of the rhythms of the upper and lower heart chambers.

HEMIPLEGIA: Paralysis of one side of the body as the result of damage to the opposite side of the brain. Nerves cross in the brain so that one side of the brain controls the opposite arm and leg. Such paralysis is sometimes caused by a blood clot or hemorrhage in a brain blood vessel.

HEMORRHAGE: Bleeding. In external hemorrhage blood escapes from the body. In internal hemorrhage blood passes into tissues surrounding the ruptured blood vessel.

HYPERCHOLESTEREMIA: An excess of a fatty substance called cholesterol in the blood.

HYPERLIPIDEMIA: An excess of fat or lipids in the blood.

HYPERTENSION: Increased blood pressure above normal.

HYPER-REACTOR: A person who reacts to even mild life stresses with an excessive rise in blood pressure. Such a person frequently, but not always, develops high blood pressure sometime in life.

HYPOTENSION: Low blood pressure. Blood pressure below the normal range. Most commonly occurs in shock.

INFARCT: Damage of a tissue as a result of not receiving a sufficient blood supply. Frequently used in the phrase "myocardial infarct" referring to an area of the heart muscle damaged or killed by an insufficient flow of blood through the coronary arteries which normally supply it.

INSUFFICIENCY: Incompetency. In the term "valvular insufficiency," an improper closing of the valves, which admits a backflow of blood in the wrong direction. In the term "myocardial insufficiency," inability of the heart muscle to do a normal pumping job.

ISCHEMIA: A local, usually temporary, deficiency of blood in some part of the body, often caused by a constriction or an obstruction in the blood vessel supplying that part.

ISCHEMIC: Lack of oxygen supply to tissue.

KIDNEY FAILURE: Uremia. Decrease or absence of functions of the kidney.

LABILE HYPERTENSIVE: Person whose blood pressure frequently suddenly shoots up for no apparent reason.

LIPID: Fat

LUMEN: The passageway inside a tubular organ. Vascular lumen in the passageway inside a blood vessel.

MALIGNANT HYPERTENSION: A particular kind of severe high blood pressure that runs a rapid course and causes deterioration of the blood vessels all over the body, particularly in the kidney.

MORBIDITY: The ratio of the number of cases of a disease to the number of healthy people in a given population for a year or other period of time. The term "morbidity" includes two concepts: (1) incidence, or the number of new cases of disease in a given population during a set period of time; (2) prevalence, the number of cases of a disease existing in a given population at a particular moment in time.

MYOCARDIAL INFARCTION: The damage or death of an area of the heart muscle (myocardium) resulting from a reduction in the blood supply reaching that area.

MYOCARDIAL INSUFFICIENCY: An inability of the heart muscle to maintain normal circulation.

MYOCARDIUM: The muscle of the heart. It lies between the inner layer (endocardium) and the outer layer (epicardium).

NORADRENALIN: Compound which produces a rise in blood pressure by constricting the small blood vessels. Sometimes used in the treatment of shock. Also called norepinephrine and levarterenol.

NOREPINEPHRINE: An important substance involved in transmission of nerve impulses and other functions of the body.

NORMOTENSIVE: Characterized by normal blood pressure.

ORGANIC HEART DISEASE: Heart disease caused by some structural abnormality in the heart or circulatory system.

PALPITATION: A fluttering of the heart or abnormal rate or rhythm of the heart felt by the person.

PATHOGENESIS: The development of disease.

PERIPHERAL RESISTANCE: The resistance offered by the arterioles and capillaries to the flow of blood from the arteries to the veins. An increase in peripheral resistance causes a rise in blood pressure.

PHEOCHROMOCYTOMA: Tumor of chromatin tissues of the adrenal glands or other areas. Can cause high blood pressure.

POLYUNSATURATED FAT: Fat, usually liquid oils of vegetable origin, such as corn oil or safflower oil. A diet with a high polyunsaturated fat content tends to lower the amount of cholesterol in the blood.

PRESSOR: Tending to increase blood pressure.

PRIMARY HYPERTENSION: Essential hypertension: common high blood pressure, not caused by kidney or other evident disease.

RENAL: Pertaining to the kidney.

RENAL HYPERTENSION: High blood pressure caused by damage to or disease of the kidneys.

RISK FACTORS: Those abnormalities known to be associated with significantly increased risk of developing a disease.

SATURATED FAT: Usually the solid fats of animal origin such as the fats in milk, butter, meat. A diet high in saturated fat content tends to increase the amount of cholesterol in the blood. Sometimes these fats are restricted in the diet in an effort to lessen the hazard of fatty deposits in the blood vessels.

SECONDARY HYPERTENSION: An elevated blood pressure caused by certain specific diseases or infections.

SPHYGMOMANOMETER: Instrument for measuring blood pressure in the arteries.

STETHOSCOPE: Instrument for listening to sounds within the body.

STROKE: Also called apoplectic stroke, cerebrovascular accident, or cerebral vascular accident. An impeded blood supply to some part of the brain, generally caused by a blood clot forming in the vessel (cerebral thrombosis); a rupture of the blood vessel wall (cerebral hemorrhage); a piece of clot or other material from another part of the vascular system which flows to the brain and obstructs a cerebral vessel (cerebral embolism); or pressure on a blood vessel, as by a tumor.

SYNCOPE: A faint. One cause for syncope can be an insufficient blood supply to the brain.

SYSTEMIC CIRCULATION: The circulation of the blood through all parts of the body except the lungs.

SYSTOLIC: Blood pressure during contraction of the heart or the force of the column of blood leaving the heart when it strikes the first big blood vessel, *i.e.* the aorta.

SYSTOLIC HYPERTENSION: Elevated upper blood pressure.

THIAZIDE DIURETICS: A family of drugs that increases the excretion of sodium by the kidneys and thereby promotes increased water excretion. These drugs are often used to combat excessive fluid retention and edema. They also produce modest blood pressure reductions and increase the effectiveness of other blood-pressure-reducing drugs, and so are often used in the treatment of hypertension.

THROMBOSIS: The formation or presence of a blood clot (thrombus) inside a blood vessel or cavity of the heart.

TOXEMIA: In general, a condition caused by poisonous substances in the blood.

TOXEMIA OF PREGNANCY: Refers to a triad of findings—elevated blood pressure, edema, and albumin (protein) in the urine—of unknown cause, occurring more commonly in the last several months of pregnancy.

TOXIC: Pertaining to poison.

TRANQUILIZING: Exerting a quieting effect; to free from emotional stress or agitation.

UREMIA: Kidney failure.

VASOCONSTRICTOR NERVE: Vasoconstrictor nerves are part of the involuntary nervous system. When the nerves are stimulated, they cause the muscles of the arterioles to contract, thus narrowing the arteriole passage, increasing the resistance to the flow of blood, and raising the blood pressure. Chemical substances which stimulate the muscles of the arterioles to contract are called vasoconstrictor agents or vasopressors.

VASODILATOR NERVE: Vasodilator nerves are certain nerve fibers of the involuntary nervous system which cause the muscles of the arterioles to relax, thus enlarging the arteriole passage, reducing resistance to the flow of blood, and lowering blood pressure.

VASODILATOR AGENTS: These are chemical compounds which cause a relaxation of the muscles of the arterioles.

VASOPRESSOR: *See Vasoconstrictor.*

VEIN: Blood vessel that carries blood from various parts of the body back to the heart.

VENTRICLE: One of the two lower chambers of the heart. Left ventricle pumps oxygenated blood through arteries to the body. Right ventricle pumps un-oxygenated blood through pulmonary artery to lungs.

# Index

# About the Authors

DR. FRANK FINNERTY is known throughout the world as a leader in the fight against high blood pressure. In addition to being a member of two national task forces in high blood pressure, he is a member of the board of directors of the Citizens Committee for the Treatment of Hypertension. He is chairman of the Therapeutics and Toxicity Committee of the Hypertension Detection and Follow-up Program. Dr. Finnerty is a professor of medicine of Georgetown University Medical Center, and chief of cardiovascular research at D.C. General Hospital.

SHIRLEY LINDE is the author or co-author of 12 medical books, and winner of The American Medical Writers' Outstanding Service Award for 1972. Her most recent books are *The Complete Allergy Guide* (Simon & Schuster), *Orthotherapy* (Evans), and *Sickle Cell: A Complete Guide to Prevention & Treatment* (Pavilion Publishing Company). She has been an officer in the National Association of Science Writers and the American Medical Writers Association, and is a public relations consultant to many medical organizations.